PRIMARY
CARE
RESEARCH

RESEARCH METHODS FOR PRIMARY CARE

The goal of RESEARCH METHODS FOR PRIMARY CARE is to address important topics meeting the needs of the growing number of primary care researchers. Purposely following a sequence from general principles to specific techniques, implementation strategies, and dissemination, the series volumes each examine a particular aspect of primary care research, emphasizing actually conducting research in the real world. The well-known contributors bring an international, multidisciplinary perspective to the volumes, enhancing their usefulness to primary care researchers. Forthcoming titles in the series will include:

1. **Primary Care Research: Traditional and Innovative Approaches**
   Edited by Peter G. Norton, Moira Stewart, Fred Tudiver, Martin J. Bass, and Earl V. Dunn

2. **Tools for Primary Care Research**
   Edited by Moira Stewart, Fred Tudiver, Martin J. Bass, Earl V. Dunn, and Peter G. Norton

3. **Doing Qualitative Research in Primary Care: Multiple Strategies**
   Edited by Ben Crabtree and William Miller

4. **Assessing Primary Care: Traditional and Innovative Ways to Evaluate Interventions**
   Edited by Fred Tudiver, Martin J. Bass, Earl V. Dunn, Peter G. Norton, and Moira Stewart

5. **Strategies for Implementing Research in the Primary Care Practice Setting**
   Edited by Martin J. Bass, Earl V. Dunn, Peter G. Norton, Moira Stewart, and Fred Tudiver

6. **Ways to Disseminate Research Findings and Have an Impact on Practice**
   Edited by Earl V. Dunn, Peter G. Norton, Moira Stewart, Fred Tudiver, and Martin J. Bass

PRIMARY CARE RESEARCH

TRADITIONAL AND INNOVATIVE APPROACHES

EDITED BY

PETER G. NORTON
MOIRA STEWART
FRED TUDIVER
MARTIN J. BASS
EARL V. DUNN

**Research Methods
for Primary Care**
Volume 1

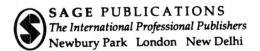

SAGE PUBLICATIONS
The International Professional Publishers
Newbury Park London New Delhi

For information address:

SAGE Publications, Inc.
2455 Teller Road
Newbury Park, California 91320

SAGE Publications Ltd.
6 Bonhill Street
London EC2A 4PU
United Kingdom

SAGE Publications India Pvt. Ltd.
M-32 Market
Greater Kailash I
New Delhi 110 048 India

Printed in the United States of America

Library of Congress Cataloging-in-Publication Data

Main entry under title:

Primary care research : traditional and innovative approaches / Peter
 G. Norton . . . [et al.].
    p. cm. — (Research methods for primary care ; 1)
    ISBN 0-8039-3870-5. — ISBN 0-8039-3871-3 (pbk.)
    1. Family medicine. I. Norton, Peter G. II. Series.
    [DNLM: 1. Family Practice. 2. Primary Health Care. 3. Research—
    methods. W 84.6 P9493]
    R729.5.G4P7373 1991
    362.1'072—dc20   90-21954
                                                                   CIP

FIRST PRINTING, 1991

Sage Production Editor: Diane S. Foster

Contents

Series Editors' Introduction

Research Methods for Primary Care is a new series of monographs on methods to understand, evaluate, and improve primary care. With the recognition that excellent medical care depends on a strong primary care sector comes a demand for data to assist primary care practitioners and for methods to evaluate their activities.

A number of factors are influencing the new methods of primary care research. Patients often present to primary care practitioners with undifferentiated problems rather than full-blown diseases. Thus epidemiology research methods require modification to be applicable. The community orientation of many primary care practitioners means that sociological survey techniques can provide relevant data but not without adjustments of their traditional format and methods. The patient orientation of primary care allows qualitative research methods to provide worthwhile insights. Therefore, although research principles and techniques can be borrowed from other disciplines, they must be adapted before they are truly useful to primary care needs.

Based on other disciplines and the evolving patterns of primary care, researchers are developing their own armamentarium of suitable research principles, methods, and techniques. This series of books reviews the present state and will support this evolution.

The series will include at least six books that are at various stages of gestation. This first book addresses three general issues in primary care research: important questions to ask, appropriate methods for different kinds of questions, and standards for qualitative and quantitative primary care research.

The second book will present tools for primary care research and will be a practical resource for investigators in need of traditional and innovative techniques to meet the unique questions of primary care. It will contain examples of basic tools such as coding schemes; sampling techniques; measurement tools, including scales and clinical assessment; data collection tools, both qualitative and quantitative; and tools for analysis.

The third book will focus on qualitative designs and techniques, which are relevant to primary care research, providing an overview of many of them. It will include discussions of participant observation, key informant interviews, deductive protocols, and hermeneutic analysis.

The fourth book will focus on methods for assessing primary care interventions whether they be therapeutic strategies, preventive programs, lifestyle changes or communications between practitioners and patients. It will stress the adaptation of existing techniques to the primary care setting.

Subsequent books will address other issues in primary care research. One book will position itself squarely where the action is, the practice of the primary care practitioner. In Canada, this is the family physician's office; in Britain the general practitioner's surgery and the patient's home; and, in the United States, the office of the family doctor, nurse practitioner, primary care internist or pediatrician. This book will provide practical guidelines for conducting research in a busy practice and how to set up networks and multi-practice projects.

Another book will address the important problem of disseminating research results in a way which will improve the quality of primary care. This surely is our ultimate goal and one which applied researchers and their partners in practice struggle to achieve. The book will provide insights into how to strengthen the links between research and practice.

The books that are presently planned in this series, and those that will be added later, will address topics vitally important to researchers in primary care. The authors will be experienced in either primary care or a number of other related disciplines and will come from not only North America but Britain and Europe.

The utility of the series of books should be apparent. The growing body of scholars in the primary care academic departments will find them valuable resources for their own growth and for teaching research methods to their trainees and colleagues. The emphasis throughout the series on *concepts, examples, practical tools* and *methods of implementation* means that the series will also be useful to a variety of practitioners (family physicians, nurses, primary care internists and pediatricians) interested in finding ways to conduct research in their practices.

We wish them well.

Moira Stewart
Peter G. Norton
Fred Tudiver
Martin J. Bass
Earl V. Dunn

Acknowledgments

The editors would like to thank the Physicians' Services Incorporated Foundation, Ontario for their generous support for the production of this volume. They also thank the Ontario Ministry of Health and the National Health Research and Development Program (NHRDP) of the Federal Government of Canada for financial support. Rudy Kremberg and Anne Stilman helped with the preparation of the manuscript. Without the tireless efforts of Marilyn Soberman this volume would not exist. Thank you all.

Foreword

The molecular revolution has evolved from a seventeenth-century linear model, aided and abetted by a concrete application in the nineteenth century known as the "germ theory." A spate of medical miracles ensued, the likes of which had heretofore been undreamed of. Medicine now has a few truly efficacious interventions for which our patients may be thankful and the medical profession proud. In all of this we have learned much about how the body functions in health and disease.

But what do we know about why our bodies adapt at some times and fail to adapt at others to a variety of external and internal stimuli? What do we know about when and where we experience life's moments of joy, fear, surprise, and sorrow in relation to our bodies' responses? Why was the patient seized with abdominal pain on Tuesday while at work and not on Wednesday while shopping? Why did another patient call for help only yesterday, instead of a week ago? Certainly genes, nutrition, toxins, barometric pressure, heavy lifting, and a myriad of other factors contribute to the web of causality. However, in addition to such predisposing, precipitating, and perpetuating factors, patients' interpersonal relations with persons near and far, real and imagined, and dead and alive, can also have important bearings on any illness. Not the least of these relationships is that with the primary care physician.

Every country that aspires to provide a health care system that is science-based, compassionate, effective, and affordable must ensure that its superstructure is founded on adequate primary care service. How else can amorphous complaints and symptoms presaging a health problem be sorted out expeditiously? How else can individuals be helped at the earliest possible moment to understand what medicine and related support services can offer, and what they must do for themselves? And who better than the primary care physician to comfort, inspire trust, and instill hope.

However, in spite of medicine's magnificent advances, we know precious little about this massive part of the health care system. For too long it has remained the submerged part of an iceberg whose true dimensions have yet to attract the attention of policymakers and the medical establishment. Apart from the public's cries for help and its resistance to the system's insatiable appetite for more money, the most effective way to illuminate problems and issues, and eventually to effect change, is through research. This is especially true for primary care.

Since the days of Robert Koch, medical research has been synonymous with wet bench laboratories. The owners of these laboratories have even arrogated the term "basic" for their particular approaches to understanding those manifestations of the human condition we call disease. What they do is assuredly of fundamental importance, but there are other approaches to knowledge and understanding that can be regarded as equally "basic."

The editors and authors of this volume have made major contributions to delineating alternative approaches to the study of that most essential of all branches of medicine—primary care. The methods discussed range from the epidemiologic to the ethnographic; they include the quantitative and the qualitative; and they illustrate the contributions of perceptive observation, accurate description, inductive and deductive reasoning, hypothesis generating, and hypothesis testing. Numerous practical examples of problems and designs are provided. Not only the patient's physical problems but also their meaning to the patient, whether as cause or effect, are seen as important for understanding the genesis of disease and supporting its ensuing course. That most potent of all therapeutic modalities, the placebo effect (and I would add its institutional analog, the Hawthorne effect) is given special prominence by Howard Brody. Too often denigrated as the residual of a well-designed randomized clinical trial ("just the placebo effect") or dismissed as an indeterminate confounding variable affecting the "controls," it can be viewed rather as the ubiquitous manifestation of hope, caring and trust—the doctor's not-so-secret all-purpose therapy. This and other matters described in this volume deserve much more investigation than they have received to date.

And where all this research can best be done—the only place it can be done—is in primary care settings. The responsibility for studying the many facets of primary care lies with primary care physicians and nurses, in collaboration with colleagues in those other "basic" sciences that underpin the health enterprise's research efforts: anthropology, psychology, and sociology. This field has been seriously neglected, and there is much to be done. The problems tackled should be "important," meaning that they should be associated with significant suffering or disability, or consume substantial resources—time, facilities, services, or money. There is no point in studying unimportant problems: Each investigation should attempt to answer a researchable question or understand a meaningful phenomenon. And each study should be feasible within the constraints of time and resources.

What follows are scholarly and perceptive discussions of approaches for making worthwhile contributions to our understanding of health and disease at the level of primary care. These approaches are necessarily diverse: Primary care research needs to utilize fully both the left-brain and the right-brain capacities of quantitative and qualitative methods. Neither alone is good or bad, right or wrong; they complement and enrich each other.

I commend this volume to both producers and consumers of primary care research everywhere. Practitioners, investigators, editors, and their readers will find it informative and inspiring. Widespread application of these methods should do much to move medicine from its seventeenth-century model to an expanded paradigm for the century ahead.

Kerr L. White

Introduction

This volume examines some basic methods that have been and can be used to study questions facing researchers in the maturing discipline of primary care research. More than just a summary of research methods, many chapters contain examples that can serve as models for readers planning studies of their own. Other chapters deal with the standards appropriate to primary care research. This material should be useful not only to investigators, but also to reviewers of grant applications and papers submitted for publication, and to tenure and promotion committees.

In the opening chapter, Dr. McWhinney, a leading thinker in the discipline, looks ahead to the next 20 years and considers the course that primary care research must follow. Dr. Howie, a practicing physician and professor of general practice in Edinburgh, considers the issue of appropriate research questions. Dr. Starfield, a pediatrician, examines an approach to answering central questions facing primary care.

The chapters by Drs. Lamberts and Bass both look at methods for studying natural history and content in family practice. Dr. Lamberts, a professor of family medicine in the Netherlands, considers the use of systematically collected encounter data and illustrates their use in studying patients who present with headache. Dr. Bass, a Canadian family practice researcher, looks at focused natural history studies and delineates their standards and use in family practice. Dr. Dunn, a professor of family medicine in Canada, presents the basic standards for analytic studies in primary care, illustrated with many examples.

Chapter 7 looks at the study of individual patients. The author, Dr. Morris, a community physician from a small town in Ontario, Canada gives examples of and standards for case reports.

The next four chapters focus on qualitative approaches to research. Dr. Helman, a primary care physician practicing in England, demonstrates the scope and the boundaries of the medical anthropological model, and gives a comprehensive overview of ethnographic methods in primary care research. Dr. Brody examines the historical reasons for the quantitative and qualitative methods to fully understand primary care. To illustrate, he includes an example of a proposed study that will employ both methods. The chapter by Drs. Kuzel and Like, primary care physicians from the United States, considers the standards for qualitative studies in primary care, drawing both on Dr. Brody's examples and on the examples presented in Chapter 11. Chapter 11, written by Drs. Tudiver, Cushman, Crabtree, Miller, and Manca, and Ms. Brown, summarizes three studies in primary care research that have combined quantitative and qualitative approaches.

Primary care research from a nursing perspective is examined in Chapters 12 and 13. Toula M. Gerace, a family practice nurse in London, Canada, examines the various roles of a primary care nurse and how those roles can naturally lead to important research questions. Dorothy C. Hall and her colleagues outline a major nursing research project presently under way under the auspices of the World Health Organization.

The volume closes with a chapter in which five of the authors, Drs. Brody, Helman, Howie, Lamberts, and Starfield, each consider how they would answer the question, "What does the primary care physician do in patient care that makes a difference?" Their responses help demonstrate the need at this time for the use of multiple methods to answer the questions facing primary care researchers.

Thus this volume is a compendium of examples, methods, and standards appropriate to primary care research. Although these are presented for the most part by primary care practitioners, the methods the authors discuss have been developed in other disciplines and are being, and will continue to be, adapted to the special needs of primary care.

Primary care is the natural evolution of an ancient tradition pervading all aspects of human society: the relationship of the healer and the patient. To study this relationship, primary care researchers will have to combine the traditional methods of quantitative and qualitative research and build on them with scientific rigor. Ideally, a single basic science for primary care research will evolve from the multiple approaches now utilized.

Peter G. Norton

1 Primary Care Research in the Next Twenty Years

IAN R. McWHINNEY

Introduction

This chapter has two themes: First, that there is a good deal of unfinished business on our current research agenda using what I will call conventional methods; and second, that different research methods must be developed—methods that can capture the richness of texture experienced in family practice. Sometimes we come across a study that produces very significant results, but we look at it and say, "Now how does that really help me? Somehow it is not what I do. It is not quite my experience."

Before addressing these themes, I want to make two general points. The first is to suggest that we get away from the qualitative-quantitative dichotomy. There are many differences between methods of research other than whether they use quantification, and to suggest that there is a strict dichotomy is misleading: Many of us, for example, use both qualitative and quantitative methods in the same study. It is also misleading to think only in terms of two methods when there is in fact a continuum, ranging from classical experimental approaches, through descriptive research, to ethnographic methods. Furthermore, becoming overly concerned with names can lead to confusion, because there can be many names used for the same method. It could be argued that it is not always necessary to give a method a name.

The second point is to challenge what appears to be a common fallacy: That descriptive or qualitative research is only useful as a preliminary to quantitative research. In other words, it is only done because it may suggest a hypothesis, which can then be tested by the experimental method. This is not so: Descriptive and qualitative research are valid in their own right, and we use them because the questions they address cannot be addressed by other methods.

Our Current Research Agenda: Unfinished Business

Using Kuhn's (1970) terminology, we might call some of this "mopping up." Three areas in which there is a good deal of unfinished business are the appropriate technology of primary care, making the implicit explicit, and the articulation of theory.

APPROPRIATE TECHNOLOGY

Appropriate technology, a term borrowed from E.F. Schumacher (1974), means using the simplest tools that will do a job effectively with the least ecological disturbance. There is so much inappropriate use of technology: to give one widespread example, the use of intravenous morphine for the relief of cancer pain when oral, rectal, or sometimes subcutaneous morphine would be just as effective. The majority of health problems can be dealt with using primary level technologies. If we are to use them effectively, however, they need to be developed, applied, and evaluated in the primary care context. The term *technology* embraces much more than the tools we use with our hands. It also includes, for example, the way we organize our practices for special purposes, such as preventive medicine or home care, and the way we use records and communication systems. Table 1.1 lists some of these technologies: old and new, preventive, diagnostic, and therapeutic.

One of the big changes that will surely occur in the next two decades is a shift toward more home care. There will have to be technologies to help us provide this care, and all of them will need setting up, describing, testing, and evaluating. We have

Table 1.1 The Technology of Primary Care

Organizational Technology

Preventive Medicine Systems
Home Care Systems
Communication Systems
- within the practice team
- between team and other agencies

Specific Technologies

Rapid Diagnostic Tests
Ambulatory Monitoring Devices
Drug Therapies
Drug Delivery Systems
Non-drug Therapies

hardly yet begun to do this, or even to recognize that there is a challenge.

MAKING THE IMPLICIT EXPLICIT

One of the most interesting developments in medicine in the past 20 years has been the development of a "grammar" of clinical method—a set of rules at the subconscious level that can be brought into consciousness when we encounter problems. There are three situations in family practice in which we have found it useful to invoke these rules. One is in the devising of strategies for the diagnosis and management of certain conditions: acute sore throat, for example. Another is for learning and teaching; we learn a lot from our own errors and we try to help our residents and students do the same with theirs. The grammar enables us to locate the error in the clinical process—that is, to say explicitly which rule has been broken.

The third could be described as the ability to refute erroneous advice. From time to time we receive well-intentioned advice as to how to act in our practices, such as "you should be doing this test," or "you should be using this treatment." Sometimes we know intuitively that the advice is wrong, but the only way we can say why it is wrong is by invoking the grammar of decision making. For example, some time ago a consensus conference of the National Institutes of Health (N.I.H., 1982) produced some recommendations on the use of C.A.T. scans in patients with headache, one of which stated that a C.A.T. scan should be done in any patient with a severe headache. We know intuitively that this is wrong, but can we say why it is wrong? What information do we need to substantiate this? First, we need information on the incidence of new cases of headache in primary care. We have quite reliable data on that. Second, we want information on the sensitivity and specificity of the C.A.T. scan. For purposes of this chapter, assume that since the C.A.T. is a good test, these are probably about 95%. Next, we need to know the prevalence of *severe* headaches in patients with this disorder. We know that this is about 50%: half the patients who present with headache say their pain is severe. The final piece of information we need is the prevalence of the target disorder—intracranial disease—in those cases. There our data are missing, or at best very sparse. It is not enough to be able to say that only $n\%$ of patients with severe headache have intracranial lesions, and that these were diagnosed without subjecting all patients to a CT scan. We have to say that all patients were followed for long enough to show that none of the non-scanned patients were subsequently found to have lesions.

This is one of the big defects of our research—that so much of the descriptive work being done in family medicine has a very short time scale. It is very uncommon to find a prospective study of the natural history of a symptom, complaint, or disease in a family practice population with a follow-up period of longer than three months. Yet this is potentially one of our strengths: We have the opportunity, particularly in personal private practice, to follow people for long periods of time. When James MacKenzie (Mair, 1973) made the very important discovery that sinus arrhythmia was an attribute of a normal heart, he made meticulous observations on his patients and followed them for 15 years. I am not suggesting that we should necessarily follow our patients for 15 years, but even one year would be an improvement. There has been so little work done on the common problems of family practice, the kind of work that an individual practitioner could do, or, for problems that are a bit less common, that a small group could do. This would not need a sophisticated knowledge of research methods.

THE ARTICULATION OF THEORY

All medicine is based on theory. In family medicine our theory is on the connection between human experience, life events, human relationships, and health and ill health. One of the items in our research agenda is the working out of the connections between these aspects of experience.

The Need for Different Research Methods

We need different research methods because some of the key questions in family medicine will not yield to current ones. For example, how do family physicians work with families? We talk and talk about this, but we do not know because so few people have studied it effectively.

Again, what does it mean to care for our patients at home? What does it mean for the patient, for us, for the relationship, and for the care that patients receive? I do not think these questions will yield to the kind of conventional methods we have been using. Indeed, using the wrong research method to answer a particular question may lead us to false conclusions.

When thinking about different ways of studying the problems we encounter, the most important thing to remember is that family medicine is a human science. What does this mean? First, human science is about *meaning*—the meaning of events, of experience, of symbols, utterances, and behavior. Second, the scope for generalization is limited: not absent, but limited. Third, context is all-important. Fourth, causal thinking applies only to a limited extent. Fifth, prediction is not a very practical objective, because prediction in human affairs is fallible. *Understanding* rather than prediction is the objective of a human science. Finally, the process of research is interactive: person to person. This is how meaning is established. It has many implications, one of them being that the process actually changes people, including the people doing the research.

In *The Varieties of Religious Experience*, William James (1958) wrote: "A large acquaintance with particulars often makes us wiser than the possession of abstract formulas, however deep." That book is based on a series of case studies and narratives of

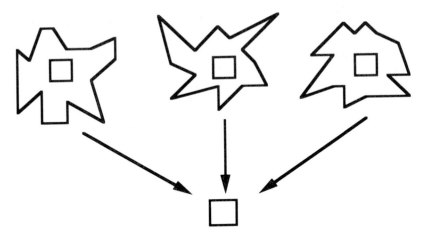

Figure 1.1. Abstraction and Generalization

various kinds of religious experience. Working from these, James was able to make generalizations, some of which have become part of our language. I suggest James's approach to psychology as a good model for us in studying family medicine as a human science.

Generalizations can be made in human science, but because they usually require us to ignore context, their value is limited. Figure 1.1 illustrates the process whereby scientists make generalizations, by abstracting from many different entities the things they have in common. In the figure, the square is a generalization. When we make generalizations we leave the context behind, and, in human science, the context is all-important. That is why abstraction and generalization may not help us very much in understanding family medicine.

Take, for example, the generalization that a poor self-concept is associated with poor control of diabetes. That is a good generalization that is in accordance with our experience. But which helps us more as clinicians: that knowledge, or the knowledge that some adolescents are so ashamed of their condition that they keep it a secret from their close friends? Or the knowledge that some parents of diabetic children will cut articles out of the newspaper that refer to diabetics so that their children won't read them, or that they wake them up several times a night to make sure they are not in hypoglycemic coma? Both types of knowledge are potentially useful, but, for myself, the knowledge that is more particular and less abstract is often the more useful in day-to-day family practice.

Every complex organic system is different: every patient, illness, and practice; every lake, river, or other natural environment; every natural or human event. With all of these, the context is important. Now this does not mean that generalizations cannot be made or that we cannot learn from studies of complex systems. It does mean however that we always have to ask ourselves: "Does this apply in my context?" It also means that research done on any human event or natural system must include a good description of the context; otherwise, we cannot answer the question, "Is this knowledge transferable to my context?"

Causality

The change from causal thinking to systems thinking is a very difficult one for those of us who were reared in the dominant paradigm of biomedical science. The successful application of the germ theory made it natural for us to think in terms of specific causal agents acting on relatively passive organisms to produce diseases. It was also natural to think in terms of a linear, unidirectional causal chain for each disease, and to regard the purpose of medical science as being to discover specific antidotes for these causes.

It is ironic that, at the same time, physicists were moving away from this simple view of causality:

> Instead of a world of passive beings waiting quiescent, independent, and unchanging, to receive an external stimulus to action from another moving body, physicists conceive of a world of permanently interconnected, mutually interacting centres of energy, whose native activity is modulated and constrained by other such centres. The immediate cause of motion is the removal of a constraint from an active material being—for example, removal of

a support from a body . . . which has an active tendency to accelerate . . . (Harré, 1981)

What we think of as causal agents may simply be acting as triggers that release some process already inherent in the organism. Whether the process is activated by the trigger depends on the state of the organism at the time. The final state of the organism, moreover, will depend less on the "causal agent" than on its own complex responses. A complex organic system does not respond to change in a simple unidirectional manner: The existence of reciprocal actions and feedback loops means that processes are circular rather than linear, and, as Gregory Bateson (1979) observed, when causal systems become circular, any event in the circle can be both the effect of a previous event and the cause of any subsequent one.

Figure 1.2 shows an explanatory model of chronic headache, based on the work of Bakal, Demjen, and Kaganov (1981). The headache begins when a causal agent, acting on a biological predisposition, produces pain. The patient's response to the pain is mediated by a belief system (the meaning of the headache for him or her). If the response is inappropriate, it may exacerbate rather than relieve the pain; this in turn will produce an augmented response, which will reinforce the headache, and so on. The original causal agent has activated a process that has become self-perpetuating and autonomous. At this stage, removing or counteracting the causal agent will not be effective.

To help the patient, we have to try to understand the whole system and how it works. Our therapeutic strategy may include several types of intervention. We may try to modify the response by using biofeedback to enrich the information flow from A to B; or we may use cognitive methods to change the belief system and give the patient a feeling of control over the symptoms. Whatever we do, we cannot be sure either that our intervention will be effective or that it will work in the way we intended. Biofeedback, for example, may work more by increasing the individual's sense of control than by actually modifying the response. Simple cause-and-effect inferences are not appropriate. In our study of patients with headaches presenting to general practitioners (The Headache Study Group, 1986), we found that the strongest predictor of resolution of the headaches at 12 months was the patient's

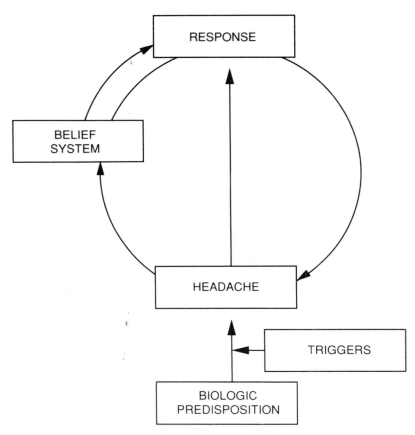

Figure 1.2. An Explanatory Model for the Mechanism of Chronic Headache

statement after the first visit that there had been a good opportunity to discuss the problem with the doctor. It is important to
understand that this is evidence of an association, not a causal
relationship. I doubt whether there is any ethical way of demonstrating a causal relationship between doctor-patient interaction
and outcome of illness; however, this does not mean that we

cannot act on this knowledge. In this type of problem our therapeutic approach is not to interrupt a causal chain, but to produce
change in a complex system. A change in one part of a system is
not limited to that part: It produces change throughout the system. If our therapeutic endeavors are directed at the belief system, we are trying to change the rules that govern the organization: That is, we are trying to change the program. One of the
distinguishing features of human science is that human beings
can rewrite their own programs, and that therapists or investigators can help them to do so.

Prediction in Human Science

All that I have said so far will help to explain why prediction
is not a valid objective in human science. In complex self-organ-
izing systems, as in human affairs, the specific effects of events
are very difficult to predict. This does not mean that we cannot
learn by studying them. We can learn from them in the same way
that we learn from history: We increase our understanding by
studying historical events and use this understanding to interpret and understand current problems, but we err if we believe
that human events ever recur in exactly the same way. Similarly,
studying another doctor's practice may help us to understand
our own or to make changes in it, but we err if we think that we
can reproduce his or her organization exactly.

Prediction in human science is also difficult for another reason.
Since human beings can "rewrite their own programs," they can,
by an act of will, invalidate any prediction we make about their
behavior.

Human Science Is Interactive

There is no empirical test for the meaning of an experience,
event, or utterance; the only way to establish what an experience
means to an individual is to enter into a dialogue with that person
from which the meaning gradually emerges. Both participants
in the dialogue may be changed by the dialogue: the investigator revising original interpretations; the subject gaining clearer

insight into the effect of an experience. The process is also circular, in that as an investigator, one has always to come back to the subject to verify one's successive interpretations.

This dialogue, also known as the hermeneutic process, is the basic element of the ethnographic method by which investigators study cultures, organizations, and institutions. The absence of empirical tests for validity obviously puts it in a different category from conventional scientific methods. It is a great mistake, however, to equate validity with empiricism. The hermeneutic method has its own rigorous canons of verification. This chapter is not the place to describe them, but they exist.

Science for Expertise: Science for Understanding

In the passage quoted above, William James said that an acquaintance with particulars often makes us *wiser* than abstract formulas. He did not say that it gives us more power or expertise. It is good to have expertise, if it is used wisely. In the past few decades medicine has shown much expertise but less wisdom. Perhaps family medicine's greatest contribution in the next two decades will be to seek the kind of understanding that increases wisdom.

References

Bakal, D. A., Demjen, S., & Kaganov, J. A. (1981). Cognitive behavioral treatment of chronic headache. *Headache, 21*, 81-89.

Bateson, G. (1979). *Mind and nature—a necessary unity*. New York: E. P. Dutton.

Harré, R. (1981). The positivist-empiricist approach and its alternative. In P. Reason & J. Rowan (Eds.), *Human inquiry. A source book of new paradigm research*. Chichester: John Wiley.

Headache Study Group of The University of Western Ontario, The. (1986). Predictors of outcome in headache patients presenting to family physicians: A one year prospective study. *Headache, 26*, 285-294.

James, W. (1958). *The varieties of religious experience: The Gifford Lectures on natural religion delivered at Edinburgh in 1901-1902*. New York: New American Library.

Kuhn, T. S. (1970).*The structure of scientific revolutions*. Chicago: University of Chicago Press.

Mair, A. (1973). *Sir James Mackenzie, M.D., general practitioner, 1853-1925*. Edinburgh: Churchill.

N.I.H. Consensus Development Panel. (1982). Computed tomographic scanning
    of the brain. *Proceedings from N. I. H. Consensus Development Conference, 4, 2.*
    National Institutes of Health. Bethesda, MD: Government Printing Office.
Schumacher, E. F. (1974). *Small is beautiful: A study of economics as if people mattered.*
    London: Sphere Books.

2 Refining Questions and Hypotheses

JOHN G. R. HOWIE

Introduction

Medicine has developed in its sophistication over the past three decades in ways none of us could have believed possible. We now have the ability to diagnose the previously undiagnosable and treat the previously untreatable, and it is research that has made all this possible.

General practice has developed, too. We have become the general physicians who used to teach us and help with the patients we could not manage. We have taken the organization of our discipline more seriously than any other professional group has done; and we have invested in teaching undergraduates and training postgraduates with commitment and effectiveness.

However, research has not "taken off" as part of our professional ethos, and there is a distinct possibility that our failure to invest sufficiently in it during the past decade, both as individuals and collectively as a discipline, will be something we will regret. Our discipline has had particularly good cause to question the benefits and drawbacks of progress. Led by Ian McWhinney (1984) and others, we have espoused the message of writers, such as Kuhn (1970), who suggest that the time has come to promote an alternative philosophy of practice to complement specialist/tertiary-care medicine. However, we are now in a scientific and professional community that wants facts and evidence both for the case for change and for the case for the status quo. We must be prepared to satisfy this demand with respect to a wide variety of issues and concepts, and sooner rather than later.

We have some very basic and easily identified problems to overcome. The first is a struggle to understand which research methods best suit the study of general practice. Although some of the researchers of general practice use conventional "medical model" techniques to answer medical model questions, an increasing proportion of our research requires "social science model" techniques to answer questions concerning the social sciences. This second kind of research may be described as "soft," but is guided by the same intellectual processes and demands the same intellectual rigor as the first. A second problem is size. Our research community is too small to supply the breadth of expertise required, and we lack the resources needed to succeed at the rate we want, and may soon be expected, to achieve.

Two things are needed. First, we need to encourage questioning, and thus research, as part of our professional way of life. The ability of general practitioners to tolerate uncertainty as a clinical skill seems somehow to have been carried too far and may be working now against our own interests. Second, we must do our best to ensure that the research we do undertake works.

Getting started is what most people who want to do research find difficult. There is no shortage of sensible and informed curiosity, but a regular difficulty lies in making the change from a situation of restless anticipation to one of effective answering. The aim of this chapter is to help bridge this gap. The first step is possibly *the* crucial one on the journey; the penalties of missing one's footing on the first stone of the crossing may only be getting wet and cold feet, but greater discomfort and discouragement are more likely, and many are swept away and never seen on the shores of critical inquiry again!

This chapter first explores what constitutes a "good question" and then looks at ways of generating a range of questions from a single starting point. At the end, I will comment briefly on the concept of hypothesis.

Defining a Good Question

Good questions always relate to experiences that are alive for the person asking them. Here is a recent clinical experience of my own that I would like to use as a running theme:

> My consulting sessions are normally booked at eight patients per hour, and I usually visit the reception area to collect each patient and sense how the place is feeling generally. When a student is working with me, the booking time is changed to six patients per hour, and between patients I discuss the consultation with the student, using the intercom to ask the next patient in. On one occasion I came to my last patient five minutes before I was due at a faculty meeting, but felt safe in the knowledge that the antic- ipated consultation on a frozen shoulder/unemployment problem would be easily accomplished. However, the patient who came in next turned out to be an extra, a drop-in, whom I had not been told about, and I had run out of time. She had dysuria. The consultation was very quick (one to two minutes), very physical in its orienta- tion, and concluded with advice to her to drink plenty of fluids while awaiting the results of an MSU culture. I felt thoroughly dissatisfied and left, only slightly late, to argue the case for more time to teach students in the clinical setting—a case I had in reality just singularly failed to honor!

Was there a research question to be created from this episode? The reader may be able to identify half a dozen without too much difficulty. It could lead to questions about the relationship be- tween dysuria and infection; about contraception and sexuality; about drop-in patients; about the effect of having a student present; or about doctors who have too many outside commit- ments, or whose orientation focuses on physical rather than emotional dimensions of patient care.

What are the criteria for a good question?

IMPORTANCE

A question must be important enough to be worth answering. It may be important because of the information it will uncover (only half of all patients with dysuria have bacterial infections), or because of more general principles that it will bring to light (the role of laboratory investigation in general practice). The question may be of interest only to the person asking it (e.g., testing my own clinical acumen against an established standard), or it may interest a group of doctors locally (What are the problems experienced in transporting urine cultures from practices to distant laboratories?) or reflect a national issue (Should use of laboratory tests attract a fee?). The scope of the research and the sophistication of the design must be measured against the uses to which the results will be put, and will be influenced by the quality of information that can realistically be gathered as the inquiry proceeds.

INTEREST

It is almost, but not quite, a corollary to importance that research should be interesting. That is not as obvious as it sounds, but it is a particularly essential attribute if the research is to require the collaboration of colleagues. I would be unable to motivate myself to join in a study of morbidity seen by different members of a group practice unless I could be convinced there was a particular benefit to be gained. Thus, in my recording of a consultation for dysuria, I would be as likely to use the inappropriate label of "urinary infection" as I would the simple descriptive term, which is more correct. I personally don't warm to studies about screening, prevention, and health education or (as may already be evident) to studies about disease classification. Each of us has our own pet likes and dislikes, which apply as much to research as to any other activity in life.

ANSWERABILITY

Being pragmatic people, general practitioners will want to see results for their research. This third attribute of a good question is every bit as important as the other two. Answerable questions are usually simple ones: Almost always if a research question is too difficult to answer, it is because several generations of research projects are hidden within it. For the individual doctor researching on his or her own, themes such as finding the cause of cancer or defining the management of hypertension are out of reach. Going back to my vignette regarding the consultation for urinary symptoms, the question I most wanted to answer was, what *really* causes quick consultations? This can be related to two more specific questions: Are quick consultations any less good than long ones? And, are quick doctors any less good than slow ones?

Peter Medawar advised us to ask the most difficult question we think we can answer. We have accepted that good questions should combine interest and importance and should be, above all, ones we believe in personally. Even the most difficult question we think we can answer is still likely to need to be a still simpler one. So, going back to the consultation for dysuria, we should now focus down a bit: Compared to doctors who work relatively slowly, do those who normally work fast (1) use investigation less for urinary symptoms; (2) prescribe antibiotics more often for urinary symptoms; and (3) explore emotional problems less often in patients presenting with urinary symptoms?

Generating Questions

Although it is helpful to recognize the criteria for a good question, there is still an often unbridgeable gap between the theory and the reality of finding the right place to start from. There are two further ways of looking at the problem:

LOOKING AHEAD TO DEVELOPMENTS

When we set a burglar alarm, the beam scans quickly across and back over the zones that the system covers before indicating that it is ready to be set. The same process should be applied in research before a prospective question becomes the definite one. Research is the process that converts a question into a numerical weighting, or statistic. This weighting either values a single numerator (an event or a measurement of an outcome or a process) with respect to a single denominator (the population of interest, described in a way that lists its key attributes and

characteristics), or compares numerator events in *different* populations (when a descriptive study then becomes an experiment or
trial).

The researcher asking a question should consider whether he
or she can first visualize and then define in words the numerator
and denominator that will be needed to answer it. The next
consideration must be whether the information needed for the
study can realistically be accessed. If the answer is yes, the
question can stand; if it is no or not sure, then either a new
question is needed or a pilot of a possible study is even more
necessary than usual.

From the vignette I have used to illustrate this chapter, I started
with a very general question: What *really* causes quick consultations? Then I moved to two ways of restating it, namely: Are
quick consultations any less good than long ones? And, are quick
doctors any less good than slow ones? I then focused on urinary
symptoms to help identify the denominator, while for the numerator, I raised specific questions about the use of investigations,
prescriptions of antibiotics, and explorations of emotional problems. With different levels of sophistication, these numerator
statements stand as provisional surrogate statements about
"goodness." "Quick" and "slow" consultations should be reason-
ably objective denominator qualities to add to "urinary symptoms." "Quick" and "slow" doctors might be more difficult,
because there are probably many who are not consistently one or
the other. We thus have a safe question about consultations, and
a riskier one (more interesting, more important, but possibly less
answerable) about doctors.

A CONCEPTUAL FRAMEWORK

I have deliberately introduced the concept of *visualizing* the
research question as a way of helping to refine it. Doctors, like
architects but unlike lawyers, are believed to conceptualize visu-
ally rather than verbally, and I find the visual refining of a
research question an essential preliminary to making a verbal
commitment to it. In the example above, I have a mental picture
of the quick or slow consultation and the quick or slow doctor,
and can quickly envisage a range of scenarios involving them. I
can also categorize many of these scenarios into "good" or "bad,"

or alternatively, as "more defendable" or "less defendable." In addition, I can experiment in my mind with ways in which I could control for certain variables (for example, time of day, or fatigue of doctor, or age or sex of patient) that would allow me to make a closer and safer study of the relationship between other variables that interest me.

Our ability to make professional decisions of any kind (whether they entail choosing research questions or responding to requests for clinical advice) depends partly on having basic knowledge and appropriate skills, but more significantly on being able to *combine and develop* our knowledge and skills in problem-solving. This in turn requires us to *analyze* problems by breaking them down into their component parts, and to *synthesize* solutions from these parts.

I am a firm believer in the advantage of having personal conceptual frameworks to help us think about any relevant aspect of our work. Most people probably have some such framework, but I suspect it is usually intuitive rather than consciously recognized. I would like to put my own framework on record here, because I use it increasingly to help solve clinical problems while teaching and, in particular, when helping others to refine *their* statements of research interests into questions.

This conceptual framework may be broken down as follows:

Part 1: I have used the term *general practice* almost exclusively, but the terms *family practice* and *primary medical care* overlap and increasingly influence our thinking about what we do. Figure 2.1 is an adaptation of a familiar diagram attributed to Horder and Horder (1954), which has been widely reused and developed. It describes in *quantitative* terms the number of episodes of illness looked after in hospital (H), in general practice (shaded) and outside the formal professional services (the larger area). It also comments on the *qualitative* relationship between patients and the health-care system, at least in relation to medicine in the United Kingdom, where access to hospitals is almost invariably through general practice. The two-way arrows indicate that people flow both ways across the boundaries, as well as in and out of the states of health and illness, and serve as a reminder that the flow is determined by complex issues that must be understood when research populations are being selected and described.

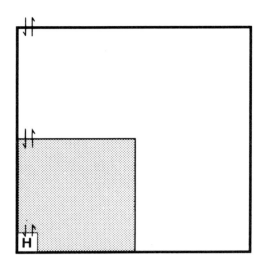

Figure 2.1. Episode of Illness Cared for in the Hospital (H), General
Practice (▓), and Outside Formal Professional Services
(white area)

Part 2: This part of my framework describes the four principal
groups of issues (Figure 2.2) that I consider when trying to
understand why a patient or other person *is* in the part of Figure
2.1 that applies at the time, and where ideally he or she should
next be.

The priority is to start with "illness" factors. These can be
subdivided into physical, psychological, and social; the physical
then divided into inflammation, degeneration, new growth, and
so on. "Patient" factors branch out through age, sex, and social
grouping into culture, health beliefs, wants and expectations, and
so forth. "Doctor" factors can be developed in the same kind of
way: Largely unexplored issues such as personalities represent a
major area for future research. "Family" issues can unite or
confound the others and may apply specifically to nuclear units,
or generally to extended families or communities.

Part 3: Figure 2.3 combines a trace of the natural history of
physical health over time with a trace of the natural history of

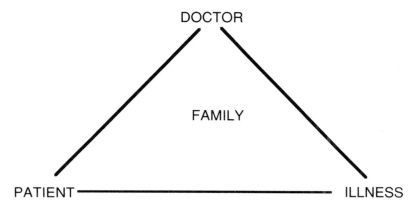

Figure 2.2. Issues in a Patient's Health

emotional health. It indicates that at any one point (say A) a physical problem may be either caused or aggravated by an emotional problem, or the relationship may be the reverse, or each may be caused by a third factor, or the relationship may be only a chance association. This, too, helps me to generate answerable smaller questions in relation to larger issues I want to explore.

There are, of course, other models. (A particularly recommended one is the much-quoted Stott and Davis [1979] model of what happens during a consultation.) The two key issues in selecting a personal model are, first, that the best model is the one the user is easily able to identify with and can therefore adapt or construct for him/herself; and second, that the model is simple. There are too many portrayals of the decision-making process that are characterized by both their extraordinary complexity and their impracticality when most needed to help resolve a real-life dilemma.

The vignette questions presented above can now easily be seen to belong to my conceptual model. Of course, I used the model to select a range of representative questions from a much more extensive possible list. If I were to decide that the issue of prescribing antibiotics for urinary symptoms were not answerable,

SEVERITY

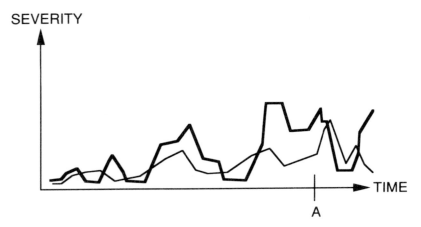

Figure 2.3. Course of Health Both Physical (━) and Emotional (—) Over Time

possibly because I would not have access to enough patients, I could revisit Figure 2.2 and the illness rubric, and might be prompted instead to switch to studying, say, new episodes of respiratory illness to determine the outcomes of quick and slow consultations/doctors. That increase in numbers might make my more fundamental question a more answerable one, and possibly make it a more interesting and important one as well. So my vignette may be best refined into a question reflecting an apparently wholly different consultation. It is this ability to look flexibly at what is the best question to research that most certainly distinguishes successful researchers from those who get stuck, lose heart, and eventually give up.

The Hypothesis

In my early days as a general-practice researcher I was still working in the "pathologist" idiom, derived from my time in academic medicine. Research was nearly always at the tightly controlled end of the investigative spectrum, experimental rather than descriptive, and usually aimed at supporting a hypothesis or disproving a null hypothesis. This model worked well in the era of more biological general practice research two decades ago, but it applies less well to the more descriptive social-science idiom that is presently the growing point of research in the community (and here I purposely do not differentiate between primary care and general practice or family medicine). So I have become less "hypothesis-centered" than I was, but I do wonder whether this is a mistake.

A hypothesis is possibly best defined (in the *Shorter Oxford Dictionary*) as "a provisional supposition which accounts for known facts and serves as a starting point for further investigation by which it may be proved or disproved." Proposing a hypothesis pushes the researcher into a commitment to trying to test the validity of a belief or even just a hunch or feeling. This is useful in that it helps determine at the outset that a particular question *can* be answered by the proposed research and, if not, whether a different design is required or a better question should be looked for.

The concept of a hypothesis brings together the various ideas this chapter explores: the criteria for a good question (important, interesting, answerable) and the ability to generate researchable questions (being able to look ahead to how the research will develop, and using a conceptual framework to help refine and select the best issue to focus on).

In the case of my vignette, I have a number of hypotheses. The most far-reaching is that slow doctors offer better service than quicker ones. But I know that this is too great a generalization to be helpful and that what is needed in the long run is the ability to describe the settings in which "quick" can be demonstrated to be less good than "slow" in a way that is likely to matter clinically. This is why I chose the specific questions above. From there I hope to open up debate on my general theme of interest, or to plan the particular way in which I personally will try to consult.

Moving from the general to the particular and vice versa is what makes clinical work a challenge and education (as opposed to training) a prerequisite to growth and development. Research is the fulcrum on which these activities have to balance. A good question is the only way into Aladdin's cave!

Postscript

Eighty-five doctors have recorded information for our research team in Scotland (which, incidentally, is truly multidisciplinary) about their work, one day in 15, for a year. At present we have information on 12,000 surgery consultations available for analysis. In summary terms, the "quick" quartile of doctors books patients at 12 per hour (and sees them at about 10 per hour); the "slow" quartile books 6 per hour (and runs later than the quick doctors). The others lie between these positions.

Urinary symptoms are the main cause stated for 2.3% of quick doctors' consultations and for 2% of slow doctors' consultations. The quick doctors sent urine for culture for 43% of their 99 consultations for urinary symptoms, as against 66% out of 42 consultations for slow doctors. Antibiotics were prescribed in 61% and 57% of the consultations, respectively, and psychosocial problems were explored in 14% and 24%, respectively.

This does not prove that slower doctors are better than quicker doctors, but, at least in the context of consultations for urinary symptoms, it is supported more strongly than is the reverse hypothesis.

Conclusion

From time to time, I have been involved in attempts to draw up lists of researchable questions and assign some kind of priority to them. As a rule, this kind of exercise does not achieve what might be expected of it: The results are usually either general to the point of being simplistic, or specific in a way that has only local relevance and is tied to a given time. I have avoided attempting this here.

I want to conclude with my favorite quotation. It is from John Berger's *A Fortunate Man* (1976), the moving and sympathetic story of the life of a country doctor. It begins with an open sketch of a rural scene, with the hint of starkness that I identify with the highlands of Scotland. There is a cottage, a hill, a field, some trees, a river, and a boat with a fisherman and his son rowing to shore as dusk falls. The text reads: "Landscapes can be deceptive. Sometimes a landscape seems to be less a setting for the life of its inhabitants than a curtain behind which their struggles, achievements and accidents take place."

Sometimes we want to ask questions about the landscapes of our work and lives; at other times we want to ask questions about what is happening behind the curtains. It would be inappropriate to give priority to either approach. There are many landscapes and many ways of looking at each, and an infinite number of ways in which we can conjecture about what goes on behind the curtains.

We can neither survive nor grow without asking questions, and I believe we survive better and grow more securely if we try to answer some of them. To find the right question requires that we understand what we are asking about, and know to keep the question simple enough to be answerable, but challenging enough to be interesting.

References

Berger, J., & Mohr, J. (1976). *A fortunate man.* London: Writers and Readers Publishing Co-operative.

Horder, J., & Horder, E. (1954). Illness in general practice. *Practitioner, 173,* 177-187.

Kuhn, T. S. (1970). *The structure of scientific revolutions.* Chicago: University of Chicago Press.

McWhinney, I. R. (1984). Changing models: The impact of Kuhn's theory on medicine. *Family Practice, 1,* 3-8.

Stott, N. C. H., & Davis, R. H. (1979). The exceptional potential in each primary care consultation. *Journal of the Royal College of General Practitioners, 29,* 201-205.

3 Innovative Ways to Study Primary Care Using Traditional Methods

BARBARA STARFIELD

Introduction

The accumulation of vast amounts of knowledge about illness makes it increasingly difficult for physicians and other health workers to know about all types of health problems. As a result, in every country, we see the tendency for health care professions to become specialized and fragmented, with the elite being those who have depth of knowledge in one field rather than breadth across fields. While this tendency toward specialization may result in care that is *efficacious*—that is, based upon the most current knowledge—it is unlikely that is will be of the greatest *effectiveness*. Why is this the case? The determinants of health are more than just medical know-how: Effective care requires knowledge of the social and environmental milieus, and these are generally not of great interest to the disease specialist. Moreover, illness cannot be isolated from the individual, and the patient is more than just an illness. Effective health care must take into consideration many aspects of the patient in addition to the illness in order to devise the most effective approach to treatment. This is the justification for providing primary care: the basic level of care that addresses the main problems in the community; provides preventive, curative, and rehabilitative services according to the problems that exist; and integrates and coordinates all levels of care that are provided over time.

The Historical Context

In 1920, in the aftermath of the First World War and eight years after the institution of national health insurance, Great Britain commissioned a "white paper" (Lord Dawson of Penn, 1920) that dealt with the organization of the health services system. This paper distinguished three major levels of services: primary health centers, secondary health centers, and teaching hospitals. Formal linkages among these three levels were proposed and the functions of each described. This formulation was the basis for the theoretical concept of "regionalization": an organization designed to respond to the various levels of need in the population. This notion provided the basis for the reorganization of health services in many, but not all countries of the world: The United States was one of the exceptions.

In contrast to regionalization, in the United States at least two coincidental phenomena led to changes that would encourage the trend toward specialization for decades thereafter. One was the rapid expansion of technology, especially after World War II, and the other was responsive third-party reimbursement, which heavily favored the use of technology and procedures. Between 1940 and 1949 the proportion of U.S. physicians who practiced as specialists increased from 24% to 37%; a trend that continued to 44% in 1955, 55% in 1960, 69% in 1966 (Starr, 1982, p. 395), and 73% in 1985 (National Center for Health Statistics, 1987). In Canada the proportion of physicians who practice as specialists has been much lower: 48% in 1986 (Minister of National Health and Welfare, 1988). Furthermore, Canadian internists and pediatricians are considered specialists, whereas in the United States, they are considered to be primary care physicians. If these two groups were included in the same category in both countries, the differences in the relative proportions would be even greater.

The concept that general internists, family physicians, and pediatricians provide primary care is a reality and allows the use of the credentials of individual physicians to define the scope of primary care. However, a substantial proportion of internists and pediatricians in the United States devote all or a substantial part of their time to the practice of a subspecialty, while in most other countries, they function entirely as specialists, providing consultative and specialized services only. It would be useful to have a definition of primary care that would make it possible to define the educational content of training programs, provide standards for the planning and design of practices, and facilitate evaluation of the adequacy of existing services. Various approaches to such an operational definition are considered below.

Current Views of Primary Care

In the 1970s a series of deliberations at the Assembly of the World Health Organization (WHO) led to an international conference on primary care at Alma Ata, USSR, in 1979. These deliberations began at the 1974 Assembly meeting, where it was noted that there were disparities in the development of health services between countries. The Director General was requested to report on what could be done to achieve more effective coordination between WHO's activities and national health programs. In 1975 the Executive Board passed a resolution that focused on primary care and its prerequisites. At the 1976 meeting the Director General presented a report on primary care and asked for an international conference on the subject (Reid, 1986). At the resulting Alma Ata conference, which was attended by 134 of the 164 member nations, primary care was defined as:

> [E]ssential health care based on practical, scientifically sound and socially acceptable methods and technology made universally accessible to individuals through their full participation and at a cost that the community can afford to maintain at every stage of their development in the spirit of self-reliance and self-determination. It forms an integral part of the country's health system, of which it is the central function and main focus, and of the overall social and economic development of the community. It is the first level of contact of individuals, the family and community with the national health system, bringing health care as close as possible to where people live and work, and constitutes the first element in a continuing care process.

By this definition, primary care is an integral part of a country's health system and the specifics of primary care will differ from one country to another.

Definitions of Primary Care:
An Empirical Approach

In the empirical approach, primary care is identified by certain characteristics of the practice. It is distinguished from secondary (consultative) and tertiary (referral) care by several characteristics. Some of these characteristics are defined below.

Primary care deals with more common and less well-defined problems, generally in community settings such as offices, health centers, or schools. Patients have direct and continuous access to the primary care service for a variety of needs, including illnesses and preventive services. Compared with specialty medicine, primary care uses less capital and labor, and is not as hierarchical in its organization. Therefore, it is more able to respond to changing societal health needs. The patient is usually known to the physician, and entry into the system is usually self-initiated, often with poorly specified complaints. The physician's major task is to elucidate the patient's problem and elicit information that leads to a diagnosis and to the choice of a management strategy. In contrast, patients who receive specialty care have often been referred by another physician who has already explored the nature of the problem and initiated preliminary diagnostic work, which the specialist then extends to obtain a precise definition of pathophysiology. Specific management is then directed at the pathophysiological process.

In contrast to specialists, primary care physicians deal with a broad range of problems, both in individual patients and across their practice population. Because of this, they are in a better position to appreciate social and environmental impacts, since they are located closer to the patient's milieu. These realities are essential to the defining characteristics of primary care practice.

From the above it is obvious that primary care practices should be distinguishable from secondary and tertiary practices by the nature of the problems encountered: the more common illnesses and more psychosocial pathology. However, at least in the United States, this is not the case. For some types of physicians (psychiatry, obstetrics-gynecology, ophthalmology, cardiovascular medicine, and pediatrics) five or fewer diagnoses accounted for 50% of visits; for others (generalists, internists, and general surgeons) this figure is 20 or more (Puskin, 1977, pp. 68-74).

Many of the conditions that are commonly seen in primary care are also common in the practices of some other specialties. On the other hand, all types of physicians except pediatricians, psychiatrists, and cardiovascular specialists have a unique "most common diagnosis" for their specialty. Thus it is apparent that neither variety nor type of diagnosis uniquely distinguishes the types of physicians who administer primary care (generalists, internists, pediatricians), at least with current coding schemes. This phenomenon may be specific to the United States, where much of the population can directly access specialists rather than requiring a referral from a primary care practitioner.

The variety of problems presented to the physician by patients varies by type of specialty. Although no particular type of problem characterizes primary care, its practitioners (family doctors, internists, and pediatricians) see a greater variety: 15 to 20 different complaints are required to reach 50% of visits, as compared with less than 10% for other types of physicians (Puskin, 1977).

Primary care practices have been assumed to have a larger percentage of visits classified as related to prevention; but, as is the case for diagnoses, the U.S. data do not uniformly support this distinction. The percentage of adult visits that are unrelated to symptoms varies from 1.8 for otolaryngologists to 61.4 for obstetrician/gynecologists, with most other specialties ranging about 10%.

Primary care practices are widely believed to involve more patients who are continuing in care. However, several studies have shown that this is not always the case. In one study (Parker, Walsh, & Coon, 1976), family medicine was the only primary care specialty that consistently ranked first in this regard, as well as in the proportion of patients who had not been referred from another practitioner. Further, this study found that the proportion of patients referred from the practice, as compared with those seen because of a referral into the practice, was highest for family medicine. Other specialties—cardiovascular, otolaryngology, and obstetrics-gynecology—also ranked high on these attributes. In summary, except for the nature of the problem presented by patients, primary and specialty care cannot be differentiated by characteristics of encounters, at least in the United States, where direct access to specialists is common.

Definitions of Primary Care:
The Normative Approach

In contrast to the empirical approach described above, the normative approach requires specification of standards of primary care and measurement of the achievement of those standards (Parker et al., 1976).

Primary care is widely accepted as being the assumption of longitudinal responsibility for the patient (that is, regardless of the presence or absence of disease); the delivery of first-contact medicine; and the integration of physical, psychological, and social aspects of health to the limits of the capability of the personnel. Such a definition was proposed in the 1966 Millis report (1966, p. 37) and is generally considered to describe the major features of primary care: *first contact, longitudinality, comprehensiveness,* and *coordination* (or integration) (Alpert & Charney, 1974; Parker, 1974).

In 1978 a committee of the Institute of Medicine (1978) listed the attributes of primary care as accessibility, comprehensiveness, coordination, continuity, and accountability. Of these, only comprehensiveness was actually defined ("ability of the primary care team to handle problems arising in the population it serves"). Accountability was recognized as a feature not unique to primary care, although essential to it. The committee acknowledged that primary care could not be defined by the location of the care, the provider's disciplinary training, or the provision of a particular set of services. However, it stated that "professionals who train men and women for primary care should accustom their students to a practice environment that meets or exceeds" certain standards, which it specified in the form of positive responses to a set of 20 questions. Seven questions were devoted to accessibility, six to comprehensiveness, four to coordination, three to continuity, and one to accountability.

The results of this committee's efforts were an important milestone in the attempt to devise a method for measuring attainment of primary care. However, there are several limitations to the checklist that was developed. First, most of the indicators might be attributes of secondary or tertiary care as well as of primary care and so are not unique identifiers: These include the opportunity of patients to schedule appointments; appreciation of a patient's culture, background, socioeconomic status and living circumstances; willingness to admit patients to hospitals, nursing homes, or convalescent homes; provision of simple, understandable information about fees; acceptance of patients without regard to race, religion, or ethnicity; easily retrievable and accessible medical records; provision of a summary of patients' records to other physicians when needed; and assumption of responsibility for alerting proper authorities if a patient's problems reveal a health hazard that may affect others.

Second, many of the indicators represent the *potential* ability to provide a service rather than its actual accomplishment. Examples include provision of personnel who can deal with patients with special language barriers, but not really providing the services to those who need it; stated "willingness" of practitioners to admit patients to other facilities, rather than the degree to which they do so when it is indicated; and stated "willingness" of the practice unit to handle the majority of patients' problems, rather than the demonstration that the unit actually accomplishes this.

Third, many of the indicators represent extreme degrees of attainment of a feature and do not allow for variability. Therefore, they may be difficult to achieve in practice; that is, they provide an absolute standard rather than a relative one.

In the long run it would appear to be preferable to develop a way of measuring primary care that is based upon the degree of attainment of widely accepted attributes, and that gauges the provision of the attribute against the needs of the population served rather than against some arbitrary absolute standard. As with the Institute of Medicine's checklist, the aim should be to facilitate self-evaluation of practice units, as well as evaluation by an outside agency, to determine the degree to which the care provided meets accepted standards.

One way to define these standards is the structure-process-outcome approach (Starfield, 1973, 1979; Weiner & Starfield, 1983). Each of the four attributes of primary care—first-contact care, coordination, comprehensiveness, and longitudinality—can be assessed by examining a *structural* element and a *process* element.

Four structural elements are required for an assessment of a primary care practice. These are similar to the indicators suggested in the Institute of Medicine report, and are defined as follows:

- "Accessibility" involves the location of the facility near the population it serves, the hours and days it is open for care, the degree to which it can handle visits made without appointments, and the extent to which these aspects of accessibility are perceived as convenient by the population.
- "Range of services" includes both the actual services that are provided to the population and which services the population believes are provided.
- "Definition of the eligible population" includes the degree to which a facility can identify the population for which it assumes responsibility and the degree to which the individuals in the served population know that they are so identified.
- "Continuity" consists of the arrangements by which care is provided as an uninterrupted succession of events. This may be achieved by a variety of mechanisms: ensuring that only one practitioner cares for a patient, or the maintenance of a medical record that reflects the care given (this could be a computer record or even a client-held record). The extent to which the facility provides such arrangements and the perception of their attainment by patients must be considered.

The two process elements that are required to describe the attainment of the attributes of primary care are *utilization* and *problem recognition*.

- "Utilization" refers to the extent and kind of use of health services. The primary reason for a visit may be to investigate the occurrence of a new problem, follow up an old one, or receive preventive services. Utilization may be initiated by the patient, be at the request or direction of a health professional, or be the result of some administrative requirement.
- "Primary recognition" is the step that precedes the diagnostic process. If problems or health needs are unrecognized, there will be either no diagnostic process or an inappropriate one. Patients may not complain of problems because they are not aware of them,

or they may complain of one thing when the real problem is another.

One of the elements of structure and one of process are required to measure the attainment of each of the four attributes of primary care. This is done as follows:

- "Longitudinality" presupposes the existence of a regular source of care and the use of that source over time. The primary care unit must be able to identify its eligible population, and the individuals in that population should obtain care from the unit except when outside consultation and referral are required.
- "First-contact care" implies accessibility to and use of services for each new problem or new episode of a problem that prompts an individual to seek health care. Regardless of what a facility states or perceives its accessibility to be, it is not providing first-contact care unless its potential users perceive it to be accessible and reflect this in their use.
- To attain "comprehensiveness" a primary care facility must arrange for patients to receive all types of health care services, even though it may not be able to provide all of them efficiently itself. Thus comprehensiveness includes referrals to secondary services for consultation, to tertiary services for definitive management of specific conditions, and to essential support services such as home care and other community resources as required. Since primary care facilities may define their ranges of services differently, each should make its range of responsibility explicit to its patient population and staff and recognize what services are called for in which situations. The staff should be able to provide and recognize the need for giving preventive services, as well as deal with symptoms, signs, and diagnoses of manifest illness. They should also be able to adequately recognize problems of all types, whether functional, organic, or social, since all health problems occur within a social setting, and many social settings themselves cause or predispose people to disease.
- "Coordination" or integration of care requires both continuity and problem recognition. For example, the status of problems that were noted in previous visits, or for which referrals to other practitioners were made, should be ascertained at subsequent visits. This recognition is facilitated by continuity (having the same practitioner see the patient on each follow-up) and by maintaining a medical record to highlight all problems.

Thus certain structural and process elements determine the attributes of primary care, and although the effectiveness of a system eventually must be measured by its impact on outcomes—that is, on health status—it is necessary first to determine whether these essential elements are achieved. The questions that should be asked to determine this include:

- First-contact care: To what extent does the system provide for easy access, both geographically and by having longer hours of availability? Does the defined population perceive access to be convenient? To what extent is this easier access associated with utilization of the facility by the population for new problems?
- Longitudinality: Do individuals defined as enrollees identify the facility as their regular source of care, and use it as such over a period of time? That is, do all visits to and referrals by the providers take place here?
- Comprehensiveness: How wide is the range of services that is offered? Is it explicit and is it understood by the population? In providing services, do the practitioners recognize a broad spectrum of needs within the population?
- Coordination of care: To what extent is scheduling arranged to allow patients to see the same provider at each visit? Do the medical records contain information pertinent to individual care? Is there an increased recognition of problems, and if so, is this a function of better records, of seeing the same practitioner at each visit, or of both?

With these criteria, professional and governmental groups may set standards for first contact, coordination, comprehensiveness, and longitudinality; decide which services meet them; and then compare these services with other forms of care to measure their impact. Relevant issues include the following: Is the attainment of a satisfactory level of first-contact care associated with increased satisfaction among patients, as well as with better problem resolution? Is coordination associated with less overall utilization, better understanding on the part of patients, increased patient participation in their own care, more rapid problem resolution, and fewer new problems? Is comprehensiveness associated with different utilization patterns, fewer episodes of new illness, or more rapid resolution of problems? Is longitudinality associated with better problem recognition, better understanding and participation of patients, and fewer days of disability and discomfort from illness? Are patients better served by a well-organized system of primary, secondary, and tertiary care than by one that permits them to choose the type of practitioner each time they perceive a need for care?

In addition to the unique features of primary care, there are several features that, while essential, are not unique. These include adequate medical records, continuity of care, adequate referral mechanisms, communication skills, recognition and management of psychosocial problems, and involvement of patients in their own care.

There are also derivative attributes of primary care: characteristics that would follow if the unique essential features were optimally achieved. Two important ones are family centeredness and community orientation. It seems self-evident that adequate achievement of the four essential attributes of primary care requires these to be in place: At the very least, to achieve comprehensiveness and coordination, the practitioner must be aware of the patient's family situation and community circumstances.

A variety of techniques has been proposed to facilitate a focus on the family in primary care. Family styles can be characterized either by a genogram, the family circle technique, or by inventories specifically designed to assess family dynamics, such as the MOOS and the FACES inventories (Saultz, 1988). Other techniques include the Family APGAR (Smilkstein, 1978), a clinical tool based on the prior demonstration that a family function index is related to secondary psychological difficulties in children with chronic illness. This tool measures adaptability, partnerships, emotional growth, affection, and resolve in a family context. The Family Health Tree (Prince-Embury, 1984) depicts clusters of problems within families in order to unmask the social genesis of problems that are manifested biologically. Although these tools may have potential, none has been systematically evaluated for effectiveness in improving family centeredness.

Community-oriented primary care (COPC) draws on the techniques of epidemiology, social sciences, and health services research to accomplish the following tasks (Nutting & Connor, 1986):

- defining and characterizing the community
- identifying community health problems
- modifying programs to address these problems
- monitoring the effectiveness of the modifications.

The application of epidemiologic methods, which provide data that are more representative than those derived from clinical practices, should particularly improve certain aspects of care. Diagnosis and management should be more appropriate because of better recognition of etiologic factors, many of which arise from social and environmental exposures. Improved "problem recognition" should also result, as more complete data make it easier to recognize new types of disorders and clusters of unusual symptomatology. Definitions of normality also can be refined to achieve more complete descriptions of those characteristics that are related to good health.

The application of social sciences techniques should improve the recognition of existing problems through understanding of the impact of social, cultural, and economic factors on health—including poverty, unemployment, and other stressful states.

The application of health services research techniques should provide a better understanding of the impact of various aspects of medical care and the relationships between components of the structure, process, and outcomes of health services.

In measuring the attainment of primary care, community orientation is considered a "derivative" feature, in that it would "derive" from a high level of attainment of the unique features. To achieve optimal longitudinality of care, a primary care program would not only define the population eligible for care, but would also insure that the population was aware of being targeted this way. This is the first functional step in achieving COPC (Nutting & Connor, 1986): defining and characterizing the community in a way such that nonusers of services are not systematically excluded. The second step is to achieve comprehensiveness by identifying community health problems. The third and fourth steps, modifying the health care program and monitoring the effectiveness of the modification, would follow directly from the preceding two "derivative" steps.

Conclusion

It is possible to measure each of the unique, essential, and derivative features of primary care. Facilities and training programs should devise ongoing or periodic assessments of the degree to which they attain these features, and either compare themselves to other, similar programs or see if they meet preset standards. Assessments of how well these features are attained might also be expected to illuminate some important differences in the provision of health services in different systems. For example, comparison of the Canadian and U.S. systems could be undertaken from this perspective.

It is unlikely that any primary care facility will attain perfect performance on all essential components, even those that are not unique but are essential, or those that are derivative. If expectations are set too high, patients will be disappointed and professionals will be frustrated. But justification for primary care need not depend upon the attainment of optimum standards: For the time being, it may be sufficient to demonstrate that the goals are better served by practitioners trained and organized to provide primary care than by those trained to focus on particular diseases or organ system. Once the measurement of primary care is accepted as a valid technique, attention should turn toward developing methods to evaluate its overall impact and that of each of its features on the health and well-being of the population.

References

Alpert, J., & Charney, E. (1974). *The education of physicians for primary care* (HRA 74-3113). Rockville, MD: U. S. Department of Health, Education, and Welfare, Public Health Service, Health Resources Administration.

Dawson of Penn, Lord. (1920). *Interim report on the future provisions of medical and allied services*. United Kingdom Ministry of Health. Consultative Council on Medical Allied Services. London: HMSO.

Institute of Medicine. (1978). *A manpower policy for primary health care* (IOM Publication 78-02). Washington, DC: National Academy of Sciences.

Millis, J. S. (Chairman). (1966). *The graduate education of physicians*. Chicago: American Medical Association, Citizens Commissions on Graduate Medical Education.

Minister of National Health and Welfare. (1988). *Health personnel in Canada 1986*. Ottawa: Queen's Printer.

National Center for Health Statistics. (1987). *Health, United States, 1987* (DHSS Pub. No. 88-1232). Washington, DC: Government Printing Office.

Nutting, P., & Connor, E. (1986). Community-oriented primary care: An integrated model for practice, research, and education. *American Journal of Preventive Medicine, 2,* 140-147.

Parker, A. (1974). The dimensions of primary care: Blueprints for change. In S. Andreopoulos (Ed.), *Primary care: Where medicine fails.* New York: John Wiley.

Parker, A., Walsh, J., & Coon, M. (1976). A normative approach to the definition of primary health care. *Milbank Memorial Fund Quarterly, 54,* 415-438.

Prince-Embury, S. (1984). The family health tree: A form for identifying physical symptom patterns within the family. *Journal of Family Practice, 18* (1), 75-81.

Puskin, D. (1977). *Patterns of ambulatory medical care in the United States: An analysis of the National Ambulatory Medical Care Survey.* Unpublished doctoral dissertation, Johns Hopkins University, Baltimore.

Reid, Sir John. (1986). Alma Ata and after—the background. In J. Fry & J. Hasler (Eds.), *Primary health care 2000.* Edinburgh: Churchill Livingstone.

Saultz, J. (1988). Family-centered health care. In R. Taylor (Ed.), *Family medicine: Principles and practice* (3rd ed.). New York: Springer-Verlag.

Smilkstein, G. (1978). The family APGAR: A proposal for a family function test and its uses by physicians. *Journal of Family Practice, 6* (6), 1231-1239.

Starfield, B. (1973). Health services research: A working model. *New England Journal of Medicine, 289,* 132-136.

Starr, P. (1982). *The social transformation of American medicine.* New York: Basic Books.

Weiner, J., & Starfield, B. (1983). Measurement and the primary care roles of office-based physicians. *American Journal of Public Health, 73,* 666-671.

4 Episode-Oriented Epidemiology in Family Practice: The Practical Use of the International Classification of Primary Care (ICPC) as Illustrated in Patients with Headache

HENK LAMBERTS

Introduction

Information systems and health statistics deal with data that have been ordered and named so that they can be counted. What has not been given a name cannot be counted, and consequently has no impact (White, 1985). The International Classification of Primary Care (ICPC), together with its manual, provides a new tool to order and name essential elements of primary care (Lamberts & Wood, 1987). It offers a comprehensive classification system, which can be used in three modes: as a reason for encounter classification, as a diagnostic classification, and as a process classification.

Comprehensive use of ICPC allows us to proceed from a prevalence-oriented epidemiology toward one that is episode-oriented (Lamberts, 1986). This shift should enable us to better analyze the transitions that diseases and health problems undergo. Such transitions may be defined as the processes of change that occur during episodes of a health problem as it passes through the different elements of health care, including all the phases and changes in status of that problem.

Data from the Transition Project of the University of Amsterdam (26,945 patient years, 78,714 encounters, 73,290 episodes)

illustrate the comprehensive use of ICPC by 41 general practitioners in 12 practices, where all encounters with all patients
were routinely registered and coded during one year (Lamberts,
Brouwer, Groen, & Huisman, 1987).

Labeling Medical Problems

There is ample indication of the need for a shift in the orientation of general practice research and patient-oriented databases
("Health services," 1985; Lamberts et al., 1987; U.S. Department
of Health and Human Services, 1985; White, 1980, 1982). While
the quantity of available information is overwhelming, its quality
and structuring often prohibit practical use. It is a paradox that
in many countries the cost of health care is considered to be too
high, yet at the same time very little information is available to
indicate which intervention for which patient at which moment
during an episode of a defined disease could be considered as too
expensive, useless, or even dangerous. Diagnoses almost auto-
matically imply medical interventions without the opportunity
to take explicitly into account the individual patient's demand
for care.

White (1985, pp. 17-20) advocates a restructuring of the classification systems used in health care:

> Depending on where you look and whom you consult, there are
> anywhere from 17 to about 3,000 and even tens of thousands of
> different labels to assign to the health problems that beset man-
> kind. For our diverse manifestations of ill health and related
> suffering, there are lay and colloquial terms, there are symptoms,
> complaints and problems, there are functional and feeling states,
> there are chromosomal, molecular and behavioral aberrations,
> there are impairments, handicaps and disabilities, there are acci-
> dents, injuries and poisonings, there are fetal deaths and "voodoo"
> deaths, and then, there are diseases . . . The basic and senior clas-
> sification, the International Classification of Diseases, Injuries and
> Causes of Death, the ICD, on the other hand has simply grown in
> complexity and heterogeneity: in trying to satisfy everybody, it
> now satisfies nobody.

Family physicians label the patient's demand for care, often in an early stage of an episode. Labeling a problem as a disease legitimizes the medical interventions that follow, while labeling it as a nonmedical problem can prohibit entrance into the health care system (Froom, 1984; Wood, 1981). Several different diagnostic categories are used (Figure 4.1). Pathological and pathophysiological diagnoses form the backbone of the medical curriculum. Nosological diagnoses hold an intermediate position, depending on medical consensus. They may be eligible for inclusion in a "higher" category once etiology and pathophysiology are ascertained (e.g., migraine, irritable bowel syndrome, schizophrenia); however, some are no longer considered diseases (e.g., neurosis, homosexuality) and are discarded as medical labels. Symptom diagnoses (e.g., headache) are important in general practice, as are functional complaints, which are related to emotions and are presented to the general practitioner with the demand for help (e.g., tension headache). Emotions and psychological and social problems are not considered medical entities: They are dealt with during consultations as problems of life (problem behavior) and not as diseases, although they form an integral part of the daily work of general practitioners (Lamberts, 1984).

Another important aspect of family practice is the frequency distribution of diseases. Figure 4.2 provides an estimation of this distribution. In addition to the frequency problem, diagnostic considerations in primary care often differ from those of specialists. The negative predictive value (the probability that a certain disease is not the cause of the patient's problem) is sometimes more important than the positive predictive value (the probability that a disease is diagnosed with a high degree of certainty). Consequently, family physicians need registration methods and classification systems that are free of the problems formulated by White, and at the same time reflect the state of the art in family medicine (Lamberts & Wood, 1987; White, 1985).

Development of ICPC

The chain of information sources in a health care system in most countries provides a prevalence-oriented epidemiology, based on the use of the ninth revision of ICD (World Health

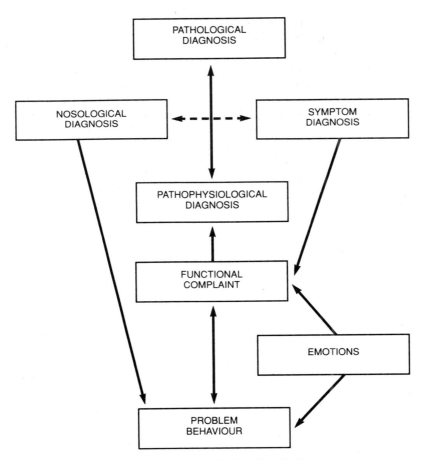

Figure 4.1. Diagnostic Categories Used in Family Practice

Organization, 1977) (Figure 4.3). However, the interpretation of the differences in prevalence, both within and between the links of the information chain, often proves to be unsatisfactory ("Health services," 1985; Lamberts et al., 1987; U.S. Department of Health, 1985; White, 1980, 1982; Wood, 1981).

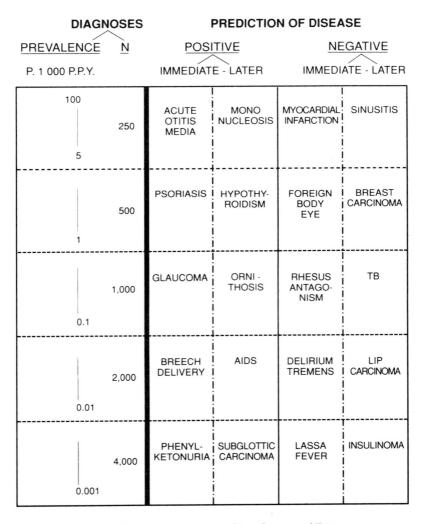

Figure 4.2. Estimate of the Frequency Distribution of Diseases as
Prevalences per 1,000 Patients per Year in the Practice of
a Family Physician

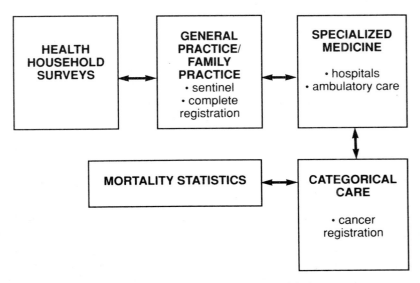

Figure 4.3. Chain of Information Sources in Health Care

The analysis of diagnosis-related information from family practice over the years has led to two conclusions:

- Numerator problems (the quality of the classification itself) tend to be underestimated, while denominator problems (the sex/age composition of the population for which incidences and prevalences are calculated) tend to be overestimated (Kilpatrick & Boyle, 1984; Wood, Mayo, & Marsland, 1986). Lack of definitions for the use of diagnostic terms and, more important, lack of understanding of the relation between the patient's demand for care and the physician's diagnostic interpretation seriously limit the interpretation of clinical data.

- Encounter-based diagnostic information is insufficient for the interpretation of large variations in prevalence of disease and the utilization of health care, both within and between the links in the information chain (Lamberts, 1986; "Variations," 1984b).

During the treatment of patients with diseases such as diabetes, hypertension, depression, or chronic respiratory disease, differences in clinical judgment between primary care physicians and specialists are not understood because we lack knowledge of the course over time (the "natural history") of diseases, analyzed on the basis of episodes (Figure 4.4). The relationships between the demands of the patient, the diagnostic interpretation by the physician, and the medical interventions that are the consequence of both, need evaluation (Lamberts & Wood, 1987).

WONCA (World Organization of National Colleges, Academies and Academic Associations of General Practitioners/Family Physicians) provides the best international forum for defining the frame of reference of family medicine, and consequently for developing and field-testing primary care classifications. ICHPPC-2-Defined and IC-Process-PC, together with the International Glossary of Primary Care, form the basis of the International Classification of Primary Care (ICPC), WONCA's latest publication (Classification Committee of WONCA, 1981, 1983, 1986; Lamberts & Wood, 1987). The ICPC system has been developed to classify simultaneously three of the four elements of the problem-oriented SOAP-registration (Weed, 1969):

S: Subjective experience by the patient of his or her problem, plus the patient's demand for care and the reason for encounter as this is classified by the provider

A: Assessment or diagnostic interpretation of the patient's problem by the provider

P: Process of care, representing the diagnostic and therapeutic interventions

O: Objective findings, cannot be classified with ICPC

STRUCTURE OF ICPC

ICPC is a two-axial classification system based on chapters and components (Lamberts & Wood, 1987). It employs three-digit alphanumeric codes with mnemonic qualities to facilitate day-to-day use (Figure 4.5). It can be used for decentralized coding with handwritten records, as well as for central coding in a computerized system. Seventeen chapters, each with an alpha code, form

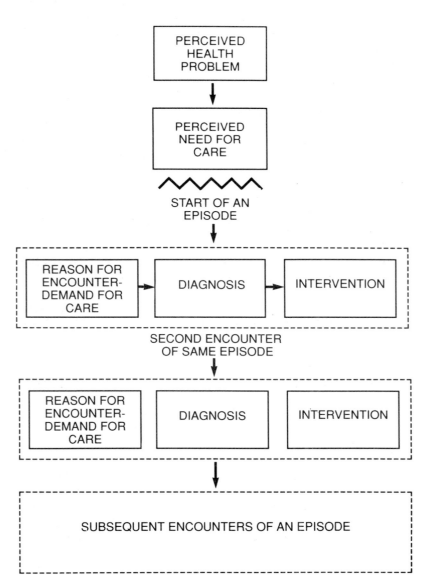

Figure 4.4. An Episode of a Disease or Medical Problem

		CHAPTERS																
		A - GENERAL	B - BLOOD, BLOOD FORMING	D - DIGESTIVE	F - EYE	H - EAR	K - CIRCULATORY	L - MUSCULOSKELETAL	N - NEUROLOGICAL	P - PSYCHOLOGICAL	R - RESPIRATORY	S - SKIN	T - METABOLIC, ENDOCRINE NUTR.	U - URINARY	W - PREGNANCY, CHILDBEARING FAMILY PLANNING	X - FEMALE GENITAL	Y - MALE GENITAL	Z - SOCIAL
COMPONENTS	1. SYMPTOMS AND COMPLAINTS																	
	2. DIAGNOSTIC, SCREENING PREVENTION																	
	3. TREATMENT, PROCEDURES, MEDICATION																	
	4. TEST RESULTS																	
	5. ADMINISTRATIVE																	
	6. OTHER																	
	7. DIAGNOSES, DISEASE																	

Figure 4.5. Biaxial Structure of ICPC: 17 Chapters and 7 Components

one axis, while seven components with rubrics bearing a two-digit numeric code form the second axis.

The system was strongly influenced by experiences with the following other classifications:

- Component 1, symptoms and complaints, drew from the experience of the National Ambulatory Medical Care Survey/Reason for Visit Classification (NAMCS/RVC) and from the results of the field trial of the Reason for Encounter Classification, which has now been replaced by ICPC (U.S. Public Health Service, 1979; National Health Survey, 1981; Lamberts, Meads & Wood, 1984, 1985; Meads, 1983).

- Components 2-6 contain the main rubrics of the International Classification of Process in Primary Care and are identical throughout the chapters (Classification Committee of WONCA, 1986).

- The classification of psychological and social problems developed by the Tri-Axial Classification Group is represented in chapters P and Z (Lipkin & Kupka, 1982).
- The rubrics of ICHPPC-2-Defined are virtually all distributed over component 7 (Classification Committee of WONCA, 1983). In ICPC, however, morphology and localization (body system) take precedence over etiology so that infectious diseases, neoplasms, injuries, and congenital abnormalities do not form separate chapters as in ICD-9 and ICHPPC-2, but are represented in component 7 of each chapter.

Classification systems are developed to order objects in classes on the basis of their relationships to each other. Identification of an object requires its allocation to the correct class (International Organization for Standardization, 1985; Sokal, 1974; World Health Organization, 1987). A good classification helps the user to:

- better define the structure of concepts;
- simplify the variations between concepts;
- facilitate memorization; and
- ease the manipulation and retrieval of data.

A concept is any unit of thought; a term is a word that designates a concept. A classification consequently arranges concepts into classes, according to established criteria. All the criteria or characteristics of a concept form its intention, while the totality of objects that have the characteristics of the concept is the extension (Nationale Raad voor de Volksgezondheid, 1988).

It is important to distinguish a nomenclature (the collection of terms belonging to the professional jargon) from a classification and from a terminology, which is based on the definition (inclusion criteria) of each term (International Organization for Standardization, 1985; Lamberts, 1987; World Health Organization, 1987) (Figure 4.6). A thesaurus is a storehouse of knowledge like an exhaustive encyclopedia or a computer tape with a large index and synonyms.

ICPC has been constructed on the following principles:

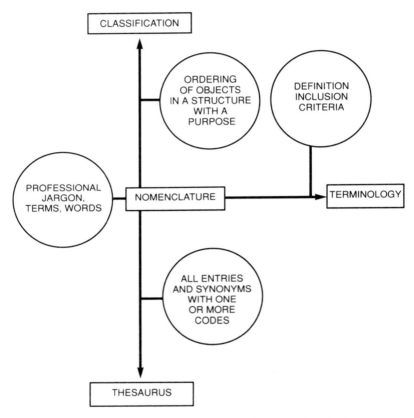

Figure 4.6. Differences Between a Nomenclature, a Terminology, a
Classification, and a Thesaurus

Concepts

- Symptoms, complaints, reasons for encounter, interventions, diseases, diagnoses

Groups

- Classes biaxially arranged over components and chapters

Criteria

- Relevance for family practice
- Localization before etiology
- Use of inclusion criteria (terminology)
- Hierarchy in specificity
- One single nomenclature for:
  - reason for encounter
  - diagnosis
  - process

A conversion of all ICPC rubrics to the corresponding rubrics of ICHPPC-2, the Classification of the Royal College of General Practitioners in the United Kingdom, and ICD-9, has been prepared and is available on tape (Lamberts & Wood, 1987). Compatibility (the ability to exist together in harmony) has been ascertained for most rubrics. Comparability (the quality of being equivalent or similar) requires a terminology, and consequently this exists only between ICPC and the defined rubrics of ICHPPC-2 (World Health Organization, 1984).

USE OF ICPC AS A "REASON FOR
ENCOUNTER" CLASSIFICATION

The reason for encounter (RFE) is defined as the stated reason for which a person enters the health-care system with a demand for care. It expresses the patient's subjective need and actual demand for care as it is clarified, understood, and classified by the provider, who responds with a diagnosis and a medical intervention (Lamberts & Wood, 1987). Many reasons for encounter are classified in the first component of ICPC (symptoms and complaints), although all components can be used. ICPC has been tested in the RFE mode for approximately 100,000 RFE's classified by more than 100 providers in 12 countries (Lamberts, Meads, & Wood, 1985). Additional studies support the feasibility and relevance of classifying the patient's reason for encounter (Lamberts et al., 1987). The reliability of coding the RFE is equal to that of the diagnosis. Its validity from the patient's point of view, however, is not known (Nylenna, 1986). Its relevance from the physician's point of view is reflected in the face validity of its relationship, or lack of relationship, with the diagnoses and interventions that are the consequence of the patient's demand for care (see Figure 4.4).

ICPC AS A DIAGNOSTIC CLASSIFICATION

In ICPC, body systems take precedence over etiology, so that chapter A (general) is the last chapter to be considered when coding a disease, which, because of its etiology, is found in several chapters. All chapters provide specific rubrics that include both etiology and the body system or organ involved.

The first component can also be used in the diagnostic mode, which allows the coding family physician a much wider scope. Formulations should be recorded at the highest possible level of diagnostic refinement, but never more specifically than can be defended by the inclusion criteria contained in ICHPPC-2-Defined (Classification Committee of WONCA, 1983).

ICPC AS A PROCESS CLASSIFICATION

The feasibility of the ICPC has been confirmed in an international field test with approximately 80,000 encounters (Classification Committee of WONCA, 1986). The structure and the major rubrics of IC-Process-PC are duplicated in the central components 2-6 of ICPC. Because the process rubrics can also be used to classify the reason for encounter, ICPC allows a broader approach to patient-oriented information.

The Transition Project

The Transition Project of the University of Amsterdam examines the relationships between the reason for encounter, the diagnosis, and the diagnostic and therapeutic interventions, together with their transitions over time (Lamberts et al., 1987) (see Figure 4.4). The model concerns complete episodes, including the influence of the health-care system on the nature and extent of the transitions. In this context, an episode is defined as a patient's health problem from the moment of presentation to the family physician until discontinuation of medical involvement, either

Table 4.1 Medical Interventions per 1,000 Patients per Year

2,680	Medical Exam
465	Lab/X-ray
1,050	Advice, Education
1,600	Medication
240	Technical Intervention
140	Therapeutic Consultation
120	Referral to Primary Care
210	Referral to a Specialist
	(Resulted in 30 Acute Admissions)
6,690	Total

because the problem is solved or because the patient or his/her environment takes care of it. The aim of the Transition Project was to gain better and more detailed knowledge of morbidity patterns and of professional behavior in family practice, on the basis of an episode-oriented epidemiological approach.

During a registration period of one year, all diseases and problems presented by all patients on the lists of 41 participating family physicians from nine practices were registered and classified. During 78,714 physician-patient encounters, a total of 120,034 reasons for encounter, 111,207 diagnoses, and 180,250 interventions were coded with ICPC by the participating physician, using self-copying encounter forms (Figures 4.7 and 4.8, and Table 4.1).

The measurement of several sources of error was ascertained in a random sample of 3% of all registered encounters. The ICPC codes for the reason for encounter, the diagnosis, and the intervention were entered erroneously by the data typist in only 0.9, 0.6, and 1.5% of cases, respectively, and miscoded or omitted by the coding physician in only 1.2, 3.3, and 1.5% of cases, respectively. In addition, only 2.6% of the encounter forms in patients' records were not entered in the database. The reliability of the information available for processing is therefore quite good.

The top 10 reasons for encounters and diagnoses at the start of episodes and during follow-up illustrate that patients' episodes

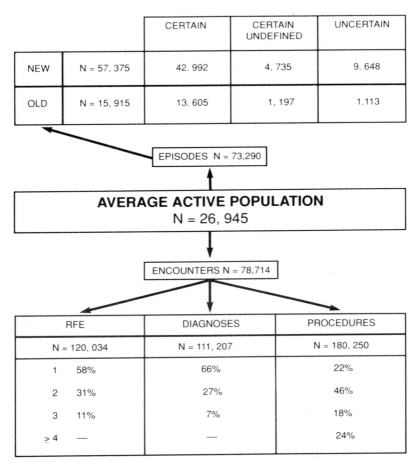

		CERTAIN	CERTAIN UNDEFINED	UNCERTAIN
NEW	N = 57, 375	42. 992	4, 735	9. 648
OLD	N = 15, 915	13. 605	1, 197	1,113

EPISODES N = 73,290

AVERAGE ACTIVE POPULATION
N = 26, 945

ENCOUNTERS N = 78,714

RFE		DIAGNOSES	PROCEDURES
N = 120, 034		N = 111, 207	N = 180, 250
1	58%	66%	22%
2	31%	27%	46%
3	11%	7%	18%
≥ 4	—	—	24%

Figure 4.7. Database in the Transition Project

began mostly with symptoms and complaints (Figure 4.9). Fol-low-up reasons for encounters were surprisingly often process-oriented (e.g., requests for examination, medication, and the initiative of the family physician). The diagnostic interpretation

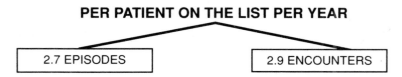

PER EPISODE
- 78% NEW
- 15% UNCERTAIN DIAGNOSIS
- 8% REFERRED TO SPECIALIST
- 4% REFERRED PRIMARY CARE
- 1% OTHER REFERRALS

PER ENCOUNTER
- 1.5 REASON FOR ENCOUNTER
  53% NEW
- 1.4 DIAGNOSES
  51% NEW
- 2.3 INTERVENTIONS

Figure 4.8. Average Utilization Per Year Per Patient on the List in the Transition Project

by the family physician at the start of episodes was primarily oriented toward acute illnesses. Follow-up diagnoses frequently dealt with chronic diseases.

Figure 4.10 shows the relative contribution of the chapters to all episodes and to all new reasons for encounter. Most reasons for encounter at the start of an episode were symptoms and complaints (component 1). During follow-up, a transition of the patient's reason for encounter occurred in the direction of the process components (requests for examination, medication, or test results). Most diagnoses were coded in component 7, but at the start of an episode the physician often used a symptom or complaint diagnosis. During follow-up there was a shift toward component 7 (diagnoses).

Headache in Family Practice

Family physicians have a great deal of interest in headache, and several publications reflect the clinical considerations in primary care. Recent publications by the Headache Study Group of the University of Western Ontario and by the Ambulatory Sentinel Practice Network (ASPN) reflect this interest (Becker, Iverson, Reed, Calonge, Miller, & Freeman, 1988; Green et al.,

TOP 10 REASONS FOR ENCOUNTERS   **NEW EPISODE (N = 63546)**

R05 - COUGH	5
A04 - GENERAL WEAKNESS / TIREDNESS	3
A03 - FEVER	2
S04 - LOCAL SWELLING SKIN	2
N01 - HEADACHE	2
R21 - S / C THROAT	2
L03 - LOW BACK PAIN	2
K31 - BLOOD-PRESSURE EXAM	2
S06 - LOCAL REDNESS SKIN	2
H01 - PAIN EAR	2

24%

TOP 10 DIAGNOSES   **NEW EPISODE (N = 57377)**

R74 - URTI	7
A97 - NO DISEASE	3
R78 - ACUTE BRONCHITIS	2
A77 - OTHER VIRUS INFECTION	2
L03 - LOW BACK PAIN	2
H81 - EAR WAX	2
R75 - SINUSITIS	2
U71 - CYSTITIS	1
S88 - CONTACT DERMATITIS	1
A85 - ADVERSE EFFECTS MEDICATION	1

23%

TOP 10 REASONS FOR ENCOUNTERS   **FOLLOW - UP (N = 56503)**

K 31 - EXAMINATION CARDIOVASCULAR	10
K 50 - MEDICATION CARDIOVASCULAR	2
W 11 - ORAL CONTRACEPTIVE	2
P 50 - MEDICATION PSYCHOLOGICAL	2
K 64 - CARDIOVASCULAR INITIATIVE F.P.	2
S 64 - SKIN, INITIATIVE F.P.	2
R 05 - COUGH	2
A 04 - GENERAL WEAKNESS, TIRED	2
P 01 - ANXIOUS, NERVOUS	1
R 02 - SHORTNESS OF BREATH	1

26 %

TOP 10 DIAGNOSES   **FOLLOW - UP (N = 53860)**

K 86 - HYPERTENSION	11
W 11 - ORAL CONTRACEPTIVE	3
T 90 - DIABETES	3
K 76 - CHRONIC ISCH. HEART DISEASE	2
R 78 - ACUTE BRONCHITIS	2
K 77 - HEART FAILURE	2
L 89 - OSTEOARTHRITIS	1
R 76 - ACUTE TONSILLITIS	1
S 97 - CHRONIC SKIN ULCER	1
R 96 - ASTHMA	1

27%

Figure 4.9. Top 10 Reasons for Encounters and Diagnosis at the Start of Episodes and During Follow-up

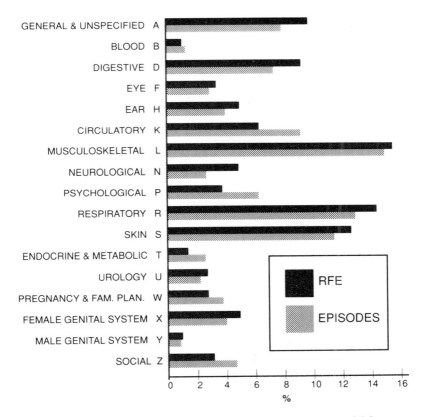

Figure 4.10. Distribution of All Episodes and New RFE by ICPC Chapter (percentages) in the Transition Project

1984; The Headache Study Group of The University of Western Ontario, 1986). In the Transition Project, headache was a prominent reason for encounter, accounting for 2% of all new episodes, which was close to the 1.5% found in the ASPN study (Becker et al., 1988). Transition Project data on patients with headache showed the characteristic transitions described above to also occur in the relationships between patients' reason for encounter, the family physicians' diagnostic interpretations, and the diagnostic and therapeutic interventions during episodes whose initial RFE is headache.

In the Netherlands, headache is a prominent complaint in health diaries: 34% of all adults recorded experiencing headaches in their diaries during a four-week period, with an average episode length of 3.2 days (Lisdonk, 1985). Fifty-three percent of the episodes were treated with self-administered medication, and in 28% of the cases normal daily activities (work, school) were limited. Only 3% of all episodes formed the reason for encounter with a physician (Lisdonk, 1985).

The Transition Project provides routine information without a specific disease orientation and without additional information relevant to particular problems such as headache. How do routine data compare with those collected in limited but more specific studies? Our study included 1,409 patients who presented with headache as the reason for encounter for a new episode, the ASPN study 1,331, and the University of Western Ontario study 272. Incidences are not available in either the ASPN or the University of Western Ontario study because the study populations were not denominated. Figure 4.11 illustrates that headache is an important reason for encounter in all three studies. It also shows that apparently quite different diagnostic criteria have been used. The inclusion criteria of ICHPPC-2-Defined apply to our study, while both North American studies use very different criteria. The main issue here, however, is not semantics or definitions; it is the question of whether a defined diagnostic entity can be linked to a characteristic distribution of reasons for encounter and interventions, thus legitimating itself on the basis of the clinical differences between the labels used.

Headache is the central reason for encounter depicted in Figure 4.12. It should be noted that nonspecific headache is one of the diagnostic categories when an episode concerns headache pain (just as tension and migraine headaches are). "Headache" will be used in what follows for nonspecific headache. In 30% of all encounters, the physicians in the Transition Project were uncertain of whether their diagnostic interpretations, following the inclusion criteria of ICHPPC-2-Defined, were correct. The use of diagnostic interventions was very modest (less than half) compared with the North American approach. Physical examination

	L01 - NECK SYMPTOMS / COMPLAINTS	L83 - CERVICAL SPINE SYNDROMES	N01 - HEADACHE	N89 - MIGRAINE	P10 - TENSION HEADACHE	TOTAL
A REASON FOR ENCOUNTER P 1,000 PAT. PER YEAR	30	—	73	3	1	107
B PREVALANCE P 1,000 PAT. PER YEAR	12	17	14	9	11	63
C TRANSITION N = 1409	3%	3%	19%	5%	12%	
D ASPN (32) N = 1331	—	—	15%	13%	24%	
E WESTERN ONTARIO (31) N = 272	—	2%	—	32%	51%	

Figure 4.11. Headache in Family Practice: Reasons for Encounters (A) and Prevalences (B) in the Transition Project and the Distribution of Diagnoses (percentages) for New Patients with Headache in Three Projects (C, D, E)

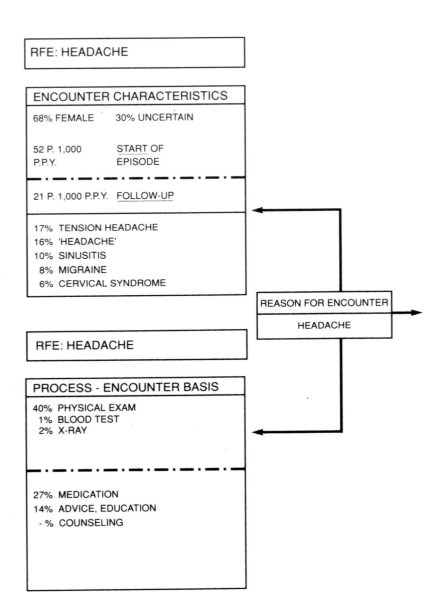

Figure 4.12. Headache as the Central Reason for Encounter

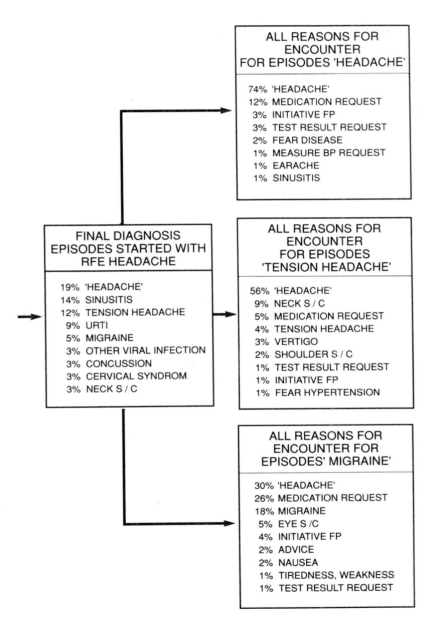

ALL REASONS FOR ENCOUNTER FOR EPISODES 'HEADACHE'

74% 'HEADACHE'
12% MEDICATION REQUEST
3% INITIATIVE FP
3% TEST RESULT REQUEST
2% FEAR DISEASE
1% MEASURE BP REQUEST
1% EARACHE
1% SINUSITIS

FINAL DIAGNOSIS EPISODES STARTED WITH RFE HEADACHE

19% 'HEADACHE'
14% SINUSITIS
12% TENSION HEADACHE
9% URTI
5% MIGRAINE
3% OTHER VIRAL INFECTION
3% CONCUSSION
3% CERVICAL SYNDROM
3% NECK S / C

ALL REASONS FOR ENCOUNTER FOR EPISODES 'TENSION HEADACHE'

56% 'HEADACHE'
9% NECK S / C
5% MEDICATION REQUEST
4% TENSION HEADACHE
3% VERTIGO
2% SHOULDER S / C
1% TEST RESULT REQUEST
1% INITIATIVE FP
1% FEAR HYPERTENSION

ALL REASONS FOR ENCOUNTER FOR EPISODES' MIGRAINE'

30% 'HEADACHE'
26% MEDICATION REQUEST
18% MIGRAINE
5% EYE S /C
4% INITIATIVE FP
2% ADVICE
2% NAUSEA
1% TIREDNESS, WEAKNESS
1% TEST RESULT REQUEST

Figure 4.12. (Continued)

took place in only a minority of encounters, X-rays were ordered in only 2%, and a blood test requested in only 1%. In comparison, in the ASPN study an additional test was ordered in 23% of first visits: 10% of these were blood tests, 4% were X-ray, and 2.5% were CT scans. Medication was prescribed in 27% of all cases in the Transition Project, compared to 74% in the ASPN study.

At the end of an episode that began with headache as a reason for encounter, the distribution of diagnoses was remarkable: 39% of all episodes were still similarly labeled "headache." Tension headache and migraine were far less prominent diagnoses, as was the case in the North American studies (Figure 4.11). The inclusion criteria used in the Transition Project were probably the main reason for this. Sinusitis, upper respiratory tract infection, and other viral infections were the diagnoses that could be compared with "febrile headache" in the ASPN study. Concussion, cervical spine syndromes, and neck symptoms and complaints were the remaining diagnoses, each accounting for at least 1% of all episodes.

The distribution of all reasons for encounter, both at the start of an episode and for follow-up encounters (displayed in Figure 4.13), were characteristic for each of the "headache," tension headache, and migraine encounters. "Headache" was by far the most important reason for encounter for a headache episode. Requests for medication, for test results, or for blood-pressure measurements were the process-oriented reasons for encounter. In 3% of all encounters, the episode was treated at the initiative of the family physician.

For tension headache episodes, neck symptoms and complaints, shoulder symptoms and complaints, and tension headache were additional reasons for encounter in visits. Requests for medication or test results made a modest contribution. The physician seldom took the initiative to discuss the problem during an encounter. For migraine episodes, the request for medication was a very important reason for encounter. In 18% of all cases, the patient's reason for encounter was migraine. Eye symptoms, nausea, vomiting, and tiredness also had a place on the list of reasons for encounters. When "headache" was the reason for a follow-up encounter, a slight shift occurred in the distribution of diagnostic interpretations: The posterior probabilities of tension headache or a cervical syndrome increased. As seen in Figure

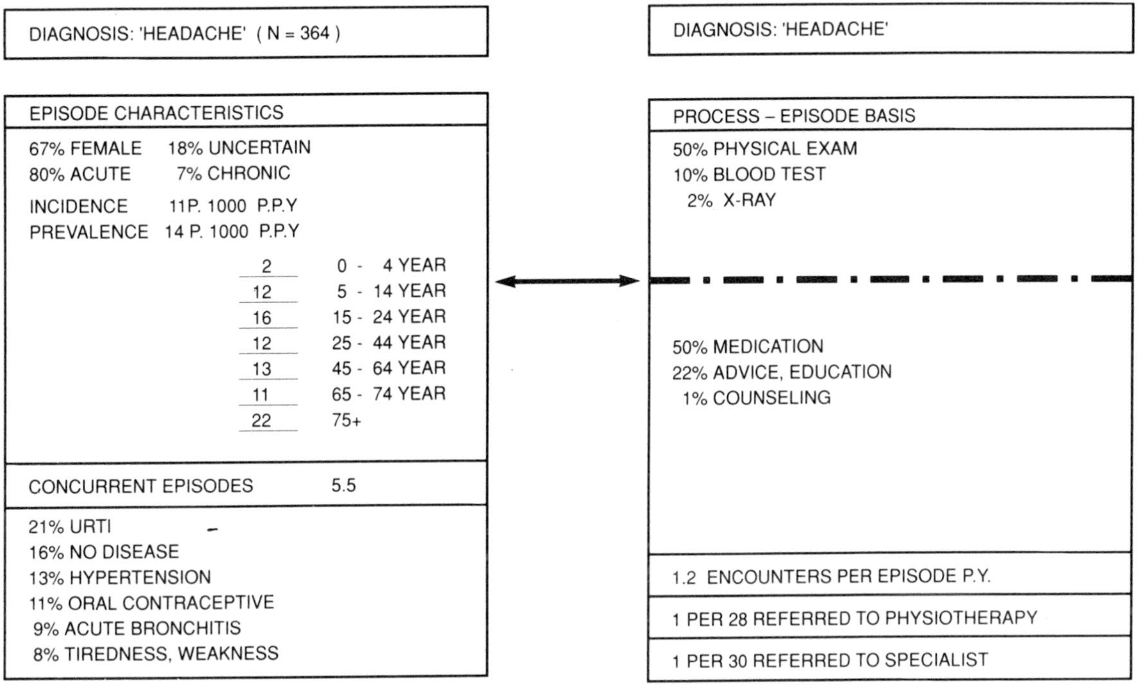

DIAGNOSIS: 'HEADACHE'

PROCESS – EPISODE BASIS

50% PHYSICAL EXAM
10% BLOOD TEST
2% X-RAY

50% MEDICATION
22% ADVICE, EDUCATION
1% COUNSELING

1.2 ENCOUNTERS PER EPISODE P.Y.

1 PER 28 REFERRED TO PHYSIOTHERAPY

1 PER 30 REFERRED TO SPECIALIST

DIAGNOSIS: 'HEADACHE' (N = 364)

EPISODE CHARACTERISTICS

67% FEMALE   18% UNCERTAIN
80% ACUTE   7% CHRONIC

INCIDENCE   11P. 1000 P.P.Y
PREVALENCE   14 P. 1000 P.P.Y

2	0 - 4 YEAR
12	5 - 14 YEAR
16	15 - 24 YEAR
12	25 - 44 YEAR
13	45 - 64 YEAR
11	65 - 74 YEAR
22	75+

CONCURRENT EPISODES   5.5

21% URTI
16% NO DISEASE
13% HYPERTENSION
11% ORAL CONTRACEPTIVE
9% ACUTE BRONCHITIS
8% TIREDNESS, WEAKNESS

Figure 4.13a. Characteristics and Process of "Headache"

63

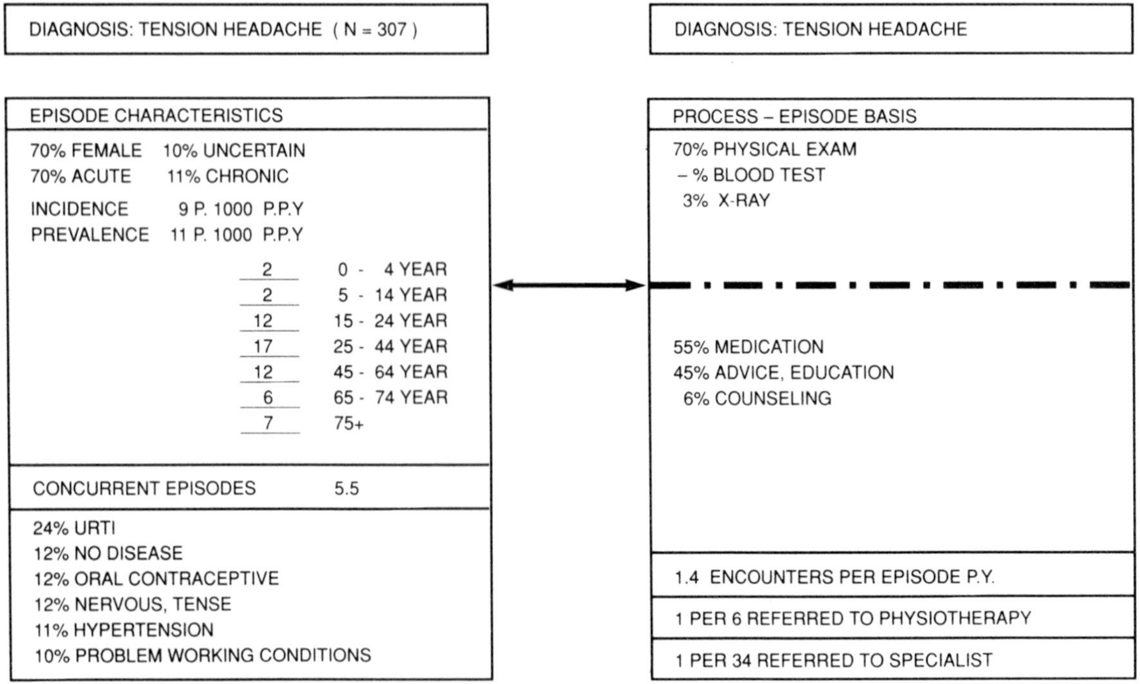

DIAGNOSIS: TENSION HEADACHE

DIAGNOSIS: TENSION HEADACHE (N = 307)

EPISODE CHARACTERISTICS

70% FEMALE   10% UNCERTAIN
70% ACUTE   11% CHRONIC

INCIDENCE   9 P. 1000 P.P.Y
PREVALENCE   11 P. 1000 P.P.Y

2	0 - 4 YEAR
2	5 - 14 YEAR
12	15 - 24 YEAR
17	25 - 44 YEAR
12	45 - 64 YEAR
6	65 - 74 YEAR
7	75+

CONCURRENT EPISODES   5.5

24% URTI
12% NO DISEASE
12% ORAL CONTRACEPTIVE
12% NERVOUS, TENSE
11% HYPERTENSION
10% PROBLEM WORKING CONDITIONS

PROCESS – EPISODE BASIS

70% PHYSICAL EXAM
– % BLOOD TEST
3% X-RAY

55% MEDICATION
45% ADVICE, EDUCATION
6% COUNSELING

1.4 ENCOUNTERS PER EPISODE P.Y.

1 PER 6 REFERRED TO PHYSIOTHERAPY

1 PER 34 REFERRED TO SPECIALIST

Figure 4.13b. Characteristics and Process of Tension "Headache"

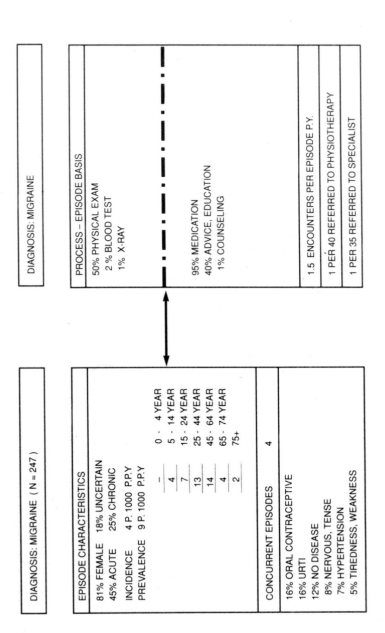

Figure 4.13c. Characteristics and Process of Migraine

DIAGNOSIS: MIGRAINE

DIAGNOSIS: MIGRAINE (N = 247)

PROCESS – EPISODE BASIS

50% PHYSICAL EXAM
2 % BLOOD TEST
1% X-RAY

95% MEDICATION
40% ADVICE, EDUCATION
1% COUNSELING

1.5 ENCOUNTERS PER EPISODE P.Y.

1 PER 40 REFERRED TO PHYSIOTHERAPY

1 PER 35 REFERRED TO SPECIALIST

EPISODE CHARACTERISTICS

81% FEMALE   18% UNCERTAIN
45% ACUTE   25% CHRONIC

INCIDENCE   4 P. 1000 P.P.Y
PREVALENCE   9 P. 1000 P.P.Y

0 - 4 YEAR	–
5 - 14 YEAR	4
15 - 24 YEAR	7
25 - 44 YEAR	13
45 - 64 YEAR	14
65 - 74 YEAR	4
75+	2

CONCURRENT EPISODES   4

16% ORAL CONTRACEPTIVE
16% URTI
12% NO DISEASE
8% NERVOUS, TENSE
7% HYPERTENSION
5% TIREDNESS, WEAKNESS

65

4.13, most episodes of "headache" and tension headache disappeared from the physician's consulting rooms within four weeks ("acute"). Only 7% of the former and 11% of the latter remained active for longer than six months ("chronic").

"Headache" as an episode had a relatively high prevalence in very old people and in patients 15 to 24 years old. The average number of concurrent episodes during the registration year was relatively high for both "headache" and tension headache: 5.5 episodes per year compared with 4 for all patients with at least one encounter during the registration year. Upper respiratory tract infections, hypertension, and oral contraception advice were important concurring episodes. Chapters P and Z, respectively, contributed 24 and 34 psychological and social concurrent episodes per 100 patients with "headache." For 100 average patients on the list with at least one encounter, chapter P contributed 24 episodes and chapter Z 18 episodes in the registration year. Thus, social problems were overrepresented in "headache" patients.

Patients suffering from tension headache consulted their family physician relatively often for nervousness and problems with work and working conditions. Chapters P and Z, respectively, contributed 45 and 50 episodes per 100 patients with tension headache, apart from the fact that the inclusion criteria required an emotional influence in any case. A strong link between tension headache and problem behavior was suggested. The significant percentage of patients with no disease reflected those cases in which the coding family physician could not diagnose a disease (e.g., administrative, check-up, advice, preventive procedure).

Migraine episodes were characteristically prolonged over time. Twenty-five percent of all episodes requested the attention of the family physician during at least six of the 12 months of registration. The predominance of women was evident, as was the relative overrepresentation of the middle-aged group. It is remarkable that in 18% of all episodes, the family physician remained uncertain as to whether his or her label was correct. The number of concurrent episodes was average. The strong concurrence with oral contraceptives can be explained by the association with the age group to which the fertile women in this study belonged. Whether pill users have a relatively high chance of suffering from migraine cannot be determined here. Berkson's fallacy, "the patient has to visit the doctor for the pill," forms a plausible explanation. Chapters P and Z, respectively, contributed 28 and 24 episodes per 100 patients with migraine, which is close to the average.

Hypertension had a prevalence of approximately 10% for all patients in the Transition Project, with at least one encounter during the registration year. Considering the age distributions for "headache" and tension headache, no indication of a positive relation between headache and treated hypertension was found.

Important differences between the three episodes exist when diagnostic and therapeutic interventions are compared. Medication was prescribed for about 50% of the "headache" and tension headache episodes. Fifty percent of "headache" and 70% of tension headache patients were examined at least once. Blood tests had only limited importance for headache. Advice was most often proffered for tension headache. Very characteristic for this episode was the high number of patients referred to a physiotherapist: one in six. Migraine was characterized by the high percentage of episodes treated with medication.

"Headache," tension headache, and migraine episodes had in common the fact that specialists played practically no part: In only 3% of all episodes were specialists involved. The percentages of follow-up encounters were limited (10-20%), which is in line with the ASPN study (21.8%).

The relationship between the duration and intensity of tension headache and the existence of psychosocial stress was an inclusion criterion, but, in addition to this the concurrence with specified psychological and social problems was much stronger than in headache and in migraine.

The use of the inclusion criteria of ICHPPC-2 for migraine resulted in the occurrence of uncertain episodes 18% of the time for migraine in the Transition Project. In the hierarchical framework of ICHPPC-2, the otherwise nonspecific diagnosis of headache is used only as a diagnosis when the inclusion criteria for the other rubrics are not met.

In the Transition Project counseling was not a prominent activity in the treatment of patients with headache: In only 6% of all episodes of migraine did the family physicians consider their efforts as a psychotherapeutic intervention. Physicians felt more at ease with the concept of a more direct approach in advising the patient on his or her daily life, explaining the mechanism of the disorder and clarifying the relations between the patient's reason for encounter, the diagnostic interpretation, and the interventions.

To summarize, the comprehensive use of ICPC, together with the inclusion criteria of ICHPPC-2-Defined, allowed for the division of headache as a reason for encounter into four important, clinically relevant diagnostic groups. Organic headache, especially in combination with febrile disease, was classified as a separate entity. Tension headache (a functional complaint) and migraine (a nosological diagnosis) could be distinguished clinically, contrary to the conclusion of the University of Western Ontario study group. The significance of psychological and social problems was quite different in the two types of episodes. "Headache" as a symptom diagnosis was found to be a useful concept, especially when the inclusion criteria for other diagnoses had not been met.

The importance of defensive behavior in distinguishing the episodes cannot be ascertained in this study. In the Monitoring Project (Lamberts, 1984), however, it was found that family physicians considered their professional behavior to be decidedly defensive in 1.9% of all encounters. This happened in only 0.6% of encounters for migraine, in 1.6% of encounters for tension headache, and in 3.4% of encounters for "headache."

Conclusion

The comprehensive use of ICPC by family physicians, who routinely register, during a full year, all vis-à-vis encounters with their patients, is an innovation in primary health care. Episodes can be characterized over time, from the start and during follow-up (Kasl, 1985). The Transition Project provides standard reasons for encounter as well as diagnosis- and process-oriented output, characterizing from three different points of view the relationships between these, both on an encounter and on an episode basis (Department of General Practice, University of Amsterdam, 1988). The available information, sometimes together with data from additional studies, is used by the University of Amsterdam's Department of General Practice in the following ways:

- as data for a free-standing research project;
- to support smaller but more specific research projects of the Department;
- as a database for the design of the medical curriculum and vocational training;
- as feedback for participating family physicians to facilitate quality assessment (Brook & Lohr, 1985);
- as a tool for expediting international cooperation in registration and classification, and for furthering the development of a standardized and harmonized approach to patient information in family practice.

The power of a large, detailed, complete, and reliable database is most helpful when questions arise that involve selection bias and pose problems with the quality of the available data. Many "realities" in medicine are not preexistent as such, but are constituted in the context of family practice when patients and physicians meet. Precise definitions of the concepts used and, above all, a better and larger terminology based on international consensus are needed. ICPC, together with the inclusion criteria of ICHPPC-2-Defined, reflects the state of the art and also provides a stepping-stone to a better system for the next decade. Routine data from complete databases will continue to form the royal route to more relevant knowledge about the content of family medicine.

The medico-cultural differences between North America and the Netherlands are considerable. Dutch family physicians simply do not consider CT scans or routine X-rays. Dutch specialists apparently treat patients with headache only after vigorous selection, because patients need referrals from family physicians. The overall pattern in the three studies, the Transition Project, ASPN, and the University of Western Ontario, is familiar: Family physicians internationally share a common frame of reference. The significant differences in the results from the three studies appear to be caused by data problems in the first place. Research in family medicine will gain enormously from the establishment of an international basis for more precise methods and better standardized and harmonized concepts.

References

Becker, L., Iverson, D. C., Reed, F. M., Calonge, N., Miller, R. S., & Freeman, W. L. (1988). Patients with new headache in primary care: A report from ASPN. *Journal of Family Practice, 27,* 41-47.

Brook, H. R., & Lohr, K. N. (1985). Efficacy, effectiveness, variations and qualities. *Medical Care, 23,* 710-722.

Classification Committee of WONCA. (1981). An international glossary for primary care. *Journal of Family Practice, 13,* 671-681.

Classification Committee of WONCA. (1983). *ICHPPC-2-Defined. (Inclusion criteria for the use of the rubrics of the international classification of health problems in primary care).* Oxford, UK: Oxford University Press.

Classification Committee of WONCA. (1986). *International classification of process in primary care (IC-Process-PC).* Oxford, UK: Oxford University Press.

Department of General Practice, University of Amsterdam. (1988). *Transition Project: Episode-, reason for encounter-, and process-oriented standard output.* Amsterdam: University of Amsterdam.

Froom, J. (1984). New directions in standard terminology and classifications for primary care. *Public Health Reports, 99,* 73-77.

Green, L. A., Wood, M., Becker, L., Farley, E. S., Freeman, W. L., Froom, J., Hames, C., Neibauer, L. J., Rosser, W. W., & Siefert, M. (1984). The ambulatory sentinel practice network: Purpose, methods and policies. *Journal of Family Practice, 18,* 275-280.

Headache Study Group of The University of Western Ontario, The. (1986). Predictors of outcome in headache patients presenting to family physicians: A one year prospective study. *Headache, 26,* 285-294.

Health services research 1984. Planning for the third decade of health services research (Special issue). (1985). *Medical Care, 23,* 377-750.

International Organization for Standardization. (1985). *Principles and methods of terminology: Draft international standard* (ISO/DIS 704). Geneva: International Organization for Standardization.

Kasl, S. V. (1985). How can epidemiology contribute to the planning of health services research? *Medical Care, 23,* 598-606.

Kilpatrick, S. J., & Boyle, R. M. (Eds.). (1984). *Primary care research: Encounter records and the denominator problem.* New York: Praeger.

Lamberts, H. (1984). *Morbidity in general practice: Diagnosis related information from the monitoring project.* Utrecht: Huisartsenpers BV.

Lamberts, H. (1986). Aan de diagnose gebonden informatie uit de huisartspraktijk; van een op de prevalentie naar een episode georienteerde epidemiologie. *Ned Tijdschr Geneeskd, 130,* 673-681.

Lamberts, H. (1987). The international classification of primary care (WONCA-News). *Family Practice, 4,* IV-IX.

Lamberts, H., Brouwer, H., Groen, A. S. M., & Huisman, H. (1987). Het transitiemodel in de huisartspraktijk. Praktisch gebruik van de ICPC tijdens 28.000 contacten. *Huisarts en Wetenschap, 30,* 105-113.

Lamberts, H., Meads, S., & Wood, M. (1984). Classification of reasons why persons seek primary care: Pilot study of a new system. *Public Health Reports, 99,* 597-605.

Lamberts, H., Meads, S., & Wood, M. (1985). Results of the international field trial with the reason for encounter classification. *Sozial- und Präventivmedizin, 30,* 80-87.

Lamberts, H., & Wood, M. (Eds.). (1987). *International classification of primary care (ICPC).* Oxford, UK: Oxford University Press.

Lipkin, M., & Kupka, K. (Eds.). (1982). *Psychological factors affecting health.* New York: Praeger.

Lisdonk, E. H. van de. (1985). *Ervaren en aangeboden morbiditeit in de huisartspraktijk.* Published thesis, University of Nijmegen, Nijmegen.

Meads, S. (1983). The WHO reason for encounter classification. *WHO Chronicle, 37,* 159-162.

National Health Survey. (1981). *Patients' reasons for visiting physicians: National ambulatory medical care survey, United States, 1977-1978* (DHHS Publication No.82-1717). Hyattsville, MD: Data from the National Health Survey, Series 13, No. 56.

Nationale Raad voor de Volksgezondheid. (1988). *Ontwerp van de WCC-standaart termen voor classificaties en definities* (88WCC09). Zoetermeer.

Nylenna, M. (1986). Open prospective recording: How is the doctor influenced? *Family Practice, 3,* 204-205.

Sokal, P. R. (1974). Classification: Purpose, principles, progress, prospects. *Science, 185,* 1115-1123.

U. S. Public Health Service. (1979). *A reason for visit classification for ambulatory care* (DHEW Publication No. 79-1352). Hyattsville, MD: National Center for Health Statistics.

U.S. Dept. of Health and Human Services. (1985). *Health services research on primary care. Program note, National Center for Health Services Research and Health Care Technology Assessment.* Washington, DC: Government Printing Office.

Variations in medical practice. (1984). *Health Affairs, 3,* 4-148.

Weed, L. (1969). *Medical records, medical education and patient care: The problem-oriented record as a basic tool.* Cleveland, OH: The Press of Case Western Reserve University.

White, K. L. (1980). Information for health care: An epidemiological perspective. *Inquiry, 17,* 296-312.

White, K. L. (1982). Evaluation and medicine. In W. Holland (Ed.), *Evaluation in health care.* Oxford, UK: Oxford University Press.

White, K. L. (1985). Restructuring the international classification of diseases: Need for a new paradigm. *Journal of Family Practice, 21,* 17-20.

Wood, M. (1981). Family medicine classification systems in evolution. *Journal of Family Practice, 12,* 199-200.

Wood, M., Mayo, F., & Marsland, D. (1986). Practice-based recording as an epidemiological tool. *Annual Review of Public Health, 7,* 357-389.

World Health Organization. (1977). *International classification of diseases* (9th rev. ed). Geneva: WHO.

World Health Organization. (1984). *International conference on health statistics for the year 2000: Report on a Bellagio conference.* Budapest: WHO Statistical Publishing House.
World Health Organization. (1987). *International nomenclature of diseases: Guidelines for selection of recommended terms and for preparation of IND entries.* Geneva: WHO-Technical Terminology Service.

5 Natural History Studies in Family Practice

MARTIN J. BASS

Introduction

The concept of physician as naturalist traces its origins to Hippocrates. There are some who claim the term *physician* comes from Greek roots meaning "student of nature" (Ryle, 1936, p. 3), so the family physician who pursues the natural history of illnesses is continuing an ancient tradition. This tradition has been given new life by Bacon (1955) and Sydenham (1848), and more recently by James MacKenzie (1920), John Ryle (1936), Will Pickles (1939), and John Fry (1966). Natural history embodies two concepts: the faithful and accurate description of the phenomena of nature, and a description of the changes these phenomena undergo over time (Freer & McWhinney, 1983).

Family physicians are in an ideal position to study the natural history of many diseases, illnesses, and risk factors. As generalists and as main providers of primary medical care, they see many illnesses in their early, undifferentiated stages; and because they provide care over time, they have an excellent opportunity to follow the courses of illnesses. Specifically, the family physician follows the courses of illnesses, and since most of our treatments are symptomatic or of limited effectiveness, this leaves much opportunity for study.

What topics are appropriate for natural history studies? Traditionally, the activity with the highest profile has been the mapping out of the natural history of a disease from its early presentation to its termination. This approach has yielded important data on prognosis and early diagnosis for infectious diseases such as chicken pox (Pickles, 1939) and recurrent tonsillitis (Fry, 1966, pp. 43-47).

More challenging but equally relevant clinically is the study of the long-term evolution of symptoms that patients present in the office. Many of these symptoms (e.g., headache, chest pain, fatigue, and memory problems) do not fit into neat disease categories, but account for much of the family physician's work. Determining outcomes, etiologies, and responses to the variety of therapies used is a theme identified by many thoughtful primary care researchers. This information is of crucial importance in managing and investigating these symptoms.

A third focus of natural history studies is the long-term follow-up of clinical and laboratory abnormalities. Just as MacKenzie (1917) determined the benign nature of sinus arrythmia, our task is to determine the significance of findings such as mild elevations of blood pressure or bacteruria. With the advent of multiple laboratory tests on the same sample of blood, we are often faced with unexpected abnormalities whose importance is unknown. The clinician, on a daily basis, encounters questions such as, "What is the significance of mild elevations of blood glucose in pregnant women?"

The most recent subject of natural history studies is the long-term follow-up of suspected risk factors. For example, the Framingham study (Kannel, Dawber, Kagan, Revotskie, & Stokes, 1961) has increased our knowledge of risk factors for heart disease and has given perspective on the roles of hypertension, cholesterol, obesity, and diabetes. The study of oral contraceptives in the United Kingdom identified both the long-term risks and advantages of the contraceptive pill (Royal College of General Practitioners, 1974).

How Can Natural History Studies Be Conducted in the Family Practice Setting?

There are two main approaches to studying the time-course of a disease, presenting symptom, abnormality, or risk factor. The first is exemplified by the very sophisticated recording system and classification described by Henk Lamberts in Chapter 4 of this volume. This type of system routinely collects data on all encounters, which then can be segmented and analyzed to answer questions about specific diseases and problems. Dr. Lamberts's analysis of the incidence and care of headache patients illustrates the power of this approach.

The second approach is to mount a specific study to answer predetermined questions. This is best done as a prospective cohort study in which the investigator has full control in specifying criteria and data collection intervals. Such an approach was used in our recent headache study, in which patients were followed for one year after their presentation in the office (The Headache Study Group of the University of Western Ontario, 1986). In this study we determined that 50% of patients were still troubled by their headaches after one year of follow-up. Factors associated with a good outcome at one year were the patient's perception of having been able to discuss the problem fully during the initial visits; an organic diagnosis; and no report of visual symptoms.

The advantage of routine data collection is that the cost is minimal once the system is running, and the data can be analyzed to answer questions that arise well after collection. The specific project approach entails the considerable expense of setting up the study, as well as the costs of monitoring. On the other hand, it allows questions that have been carefully formulated to be answered in depth.

What Is the Role of Routine Data Collection Using the International Classification of Primary Care?

Dr. Lamberts's chapter describes an impressive system, which requires highly motivated and trained physicians and constant monitoring. The results provide details about Dutch general practice that we would all desire for our own settings. In addition, the detailed information has raised exciting clinical questions for further study.

Key to the effective functioning of any data collection system is an accepted and relevant classification system. The ICPC is the culmination of 20 years of work. In Kerr White's words (1988), it deals with the problems of the living rather than those of the dead and dying. In conjunction with the WONCA definitions for problems in primary care, a powerful link in the research chain has been put in place.

The routine collection of encounter data has two main weaknesses for natural history research. The first is the reliance on the doctor as the sole source of information. This provides little information on patient perceptions, fears, or motivations. Quality of life, which by definition is measured through the patient's perceptions, can be obtained only by specially mounted studies.

The second weakness of encounter data as the main source of information is the absence of standard follow-up intervals and assured outcome data. If a patient does not return for follow-up, it is uncertain whether the problem has been resolved, the patient has lost confidence in the physician's ability to further help the problem, or the patient is coping. A targeted effort is necessary to provide this type of outcome data, which is essential for prognostic studies. Also, encounter data are tied to visits that depend on clinical needs. Natural history research often requires data on all relevant subjects at predetermined points.

Conclusion

Natural history studies are important in furthering our understanding of the illnesses, diseases, abnormalities, and risk factors that we see in family practice. Each of the two major approaches to data collection has its appropriate role.

Routine encounter data, together with the use of a powerful classification such as ICPC, will tell much about health care delivery, patterns of practice, and the common problems of family practice. Specially mounted cohort studies will provide in-depth information and insights concerning prognostic factors, outcomes and patient perceptions.

References

Bacon, F. (1955). *Selected writings*. New York: Random House.

Freer, C. B., & McWhinney, I. R. (1983). The natural history of disease. In R. Taylor (Ed.), *Family medicine* (pp. 97-104). New York: Springer-Verlag.

Fry, J. (1966). *Profiles of disease: A study in the natural history of common diseases*. Edinburgh: E&S Livingstone Ltd.

Headache Study Group of The University of Western Ontario, The. (1986). Predictors of outcome in headache patients presenting to family physicians—a one year prospective study. *Headache, 26*, 285-294.

Kannel, W., Dawber, T., Kagan, A., Revotskie, N., & Stokes, J. (1961). Factors of risk in the development of coronary heart disease: Six yeaι follow-up experience. The Framingham study. *Annals of Internal Medicine, 55*, 33-43.

MacKenzie, J. (1917). *Principles of diagnosis and treatment in heart affections*. London: Oxford University Press.

MacKenzie, J. (1920). *Symptoms and their interpretation*. London: Shaw and Sons.

Pickles, W. (1939). *Epidemiology in country practice*. Baltimore: Williams and Wilkins.

Royal College of General Practitioners. (1974). *Oral contraceptives and health*. London: Pitman Medical.

Ryle, J. (1936). *The natural history of disease*. London: Oxford University Press.

Sydenham, T. (1848). *The works of Thomas Sydenham, M.D.* (R.G. Latham, Trans.) (Vol. 1.) London: Sydenham Society.

White, K. L. (1988). Computers, epidemiology and general practice. *Lancet, 2*, 1493.

6 Basic Standards for Analytic Studies in Primary Care Research

EARL V. DUNN

Introduction

Prior to the twentieth century most studies of disease and illness were descriptive in nature and were conducted in the ambulatory setting. More recently, many of the major advances in understanding disease processes and much of the knowledge about illness and patient management have come from experiments studying patients in hospitals or institutional settings. If accurate knowledge of the diagnosis, management, and prognosis of illness and disease in the community is important, it will be essential to conduct studies in primary care settings or in the community itself.

Primary care research in the office setting can be complex, as patient problems are often multiple and undifferentiated and many conditions are seen infrequently in any one practice. Still, for primary care research studies to contribute to medical knowledge, they must meet specific standards as rigorous as those applied to other settings. These do not at present exist: As Feinstein (1989) has pointed out, "There are no standards in primary care research. . . . We will have to develop them." Although there is much truth in this assertion, there do exist standards that researchers would agree should be met for an analytic study to be considered a valid contribution to the literature. Because primary care research is a new field, the traditional research standards from the fields of epidemiology, clinical epidemiology, and biostatistics have not yet been adapted to meet the reality of its needs. Primary care researchers must understand the importance and limitations of the underlying assumptions of designs in these other fields and borrow and modify those standards that are appropriate for their own setting. Studies of methods must be done to compare new and innovative designs with traditional ones.

In this chapter, based on the existing principles for analytic studies, we give an outline of standards that we feel are reasonable, practical, and necessary in primary care. For our purposes, analytic studies are defined as those that investigate a hypothesized association or a causal relationship between factors. This definition excludes descriptive studies that do not relate two or more variables, or those that are solely hypothesis-generating. Three types of observational studies are considered here: cross-sectional, case-control, and cohort; intervention trials, both randomized and non-randomized, are considered as well. These various types of designs are described in detail below.

This discussion of standards is considered under five general headings: (1) stating hypotheses, (2) enhancing generalizability, (3) choosing an appropriate design, (4) ensuring the objectivity of measures, and, (5) drawing justified interpretations. Basic standards for each of these domains will be defined, and the major principles in each area illustrated with an example relevant to primary care research.

Stating Hypotheses

Focusing on a hypothesis is valuable because the important variables are thereby defined; confounding variables can be identified and dealt with; and appropriate statistical testing can be accomplished. Three standards should be considered here: (1) all analytic studies require at least one hypothesis, (2) all hypotheses should be testable, and (3) it is unreasonable to expect to successfully test many hypotheses in a single study.

Probably the most important decision that has to be made in any research project is deciding on the question to ask and expressing it in specific terms. This sounds simple, but in fact if done properly, can take considerable time. All analytic studies must have at least one hypothesis, or they are simply "fishing expeditions." Hypotheses must have a clear and focused outcome that in most cases will result in a discrete number or a dichotomous answer (yes or no). A project with too many hypotheses is usually too ambitious or is not well thought out. If there are more than 20 independent hypotheses (outcomes), then at least one of them will probably be significant at the 0.05 level purely by chance. The number of hypotheses that is reasonable for a given study relates to the study design, the sample size, and the statistical techniques to be used. If you are unsure about any of these, consult a statistician before you start. Most important, keep your hypothesis and study as simple as possible.

EXAMPLE

A busy family practitioner became fascinated with the data in his obstetrical practice. To better understand what was happening, he developed a form that collected data on many aspects of his prenatal care, the health of the newborn, the mother's status, and any complications of pregnancy, delivery, and the postpartum period. After three years he had collected more than 400 cases with nearly 200 variables for each. He then asked a consultant for advice as to how he might analyze his data.

This physician had become interested in one of the most common questions of primary care practitioners: "How am I doing?" He had developed an instrument to collect data and had spent precious hours collecting and verifying them. But what was his question (hypothesis)? He had none! What were his outcomes? He had none! Now that he has completed his data collection, what can he and his consultant do? The data would probably make a good database for a description of his particular practice, but the findings cannot be generalized, so further analysis is probably not justified. At best, he may be able to use them to propose hypotheses that could then be tested properly. Ultimately, he is very disappointed—after spending a lot of time, effort, and thought on this project, he has little to show for it. This type of approach, unfortunately, is all too common.

What might have been done differently to develop a good research project and, at the same time, satisfy this physician's desire to document his obstetrical care and its outcome? Before designing his form and starting to collect data, he should have developed one or more hypotheses. One appropriate question to ask might have been whether the use of this form by family physicians would result in better obstetrical outcomes, as measured by newborn birth weight. He could then have randomly assigned patients to have the form completed or not. If there was a clinically significant difference related to the form, after about 200 patients he would probably have been able to detect this, and in addition would have obtained the descriptive data he wanted. Such a project might have made a genuine contribution to basic knowledge in primary care, and his time and effort would have been rewarded.

Enhancing Generalizability (External Validity)

To enhance the generalizability of analytic studies, four basic standards must be considered: (1) the study population must be defined, (2) the need for an unbiased selection process should be assessed, (3) inclusions and exclusions must be stated explicitly, and (4) a clear definition of terms must be made.

Ideally, to generalize the findings of a research study, the study sample must be either the total (well defined) population, or a sample randomly drawn from it. The sample is not of interest in its own right, but for what it tells about the population. A careful description of the population (and of the setting) is required. This can be a problem in primary care, where, for example, a physician may not really know which patients consider him or her to be their family doctor.

At a minimum, a description of the population in terms of age/sex distribution, education levels, income, and other relevant demographics is recommended, since generalizations can only be made to the population from which the sample was derived. Does the setting include the whole community, the population of sick persons, or visitors to one or more health facilities? Too often, studies that advocate new treatments or diagnostic tests in primary care are done in tertiary care facilities on a highly selected patient population. And, just as it is usually not valid to generalize from a specialty hospital setting to primary medical care, the same holds for generalizing from the office setting to the community.

When statistical analysis will be used to generalize from a sample to a broader population, the best sampling technique is random selection, as this gives each individual in the population an equal probability of being part of the sample. There are a number of accepted random sampling methods, each with its own limitations: simple, stratified, multi-stage, and cluster. Departures from randomization introduce a bias and must be accounted for in the report; and in some cases, they may invalidate the results. To test the success of the selection process, comparisons of the demographics of the groups should be carried out.

However, the ideal situation described above is often not possible in the primary care setting for three reasons. First, lack of accurate knowledge of practice populations, as was pointed out above, is a major obstacle. Second, many conditions that primary care researchers wish to study have low prevalence; thus, to include sufficient subjects in the study the investigator must take them "as they come" and has, at best, a vague idea of the population that these subjects represent. Third, primary care providers are typically very busy, and when they are involved in research, whether as main investigators or as collaborators, their time is at a premium. Consequently, subject recruitment must be convenient, which works against random selection. Sometimes these obstacles can be overcome, but often they must be lived with. In the latter case, the recruitment biases must be reported, as well as the strengths and weaknesses that the selection process lends to the final interpretation of the findings. Future methodological investigation is needed in the area of subject selection in primary care research.

To assist in later generalization, subject inclusion and exclusion criteria must be stated explicitly, including those applied to selection from the population and those applied to allocation to intervention groups. Consideration must be given to hidden exclusions, such as the illiterate or those who speak a different language. The basic demographics of all subjects who declined to participate or were lost to follow-up must also be identified and considered in subsequent analysis.

All terms that describe the conditions used to select or allocate subjects or to assign outcomes must be defined and, where possible, should be the accepted standard definitions. This includes demographic variables such as income or social status; diagnostic labels; and outcomes such as morbidity or mortality. For diagnoses, developed classification systems such as those described in Chapter 4 are useful and allow the comparison of results across studies.

EXAMPLE

Several family physicians in southern Ontario cooperated in developing and conducting a study of headache (The Headache Study Group, 1986). They studied all patients who visited their offices over a period of one year, collecting data on the types and frequency of headaches and the factors that might be associated with problem resolution after this period. In preparing their results for publication, they considered to what extent they could generalize their findings.

A number of questions arise. How representative are these physicians of all those practicing in southern Ontario, in all of Ontario, in Canada, in North America? (Physicians who volunteer to participate in research studies are not necessarily a representative sample.) What is the age/sex distribution and the education and income levels of their patients? (All these variables can be compared with those of the general population of Ontario to ascertain how closely the sample matches the average for the province.) Since the data are all from visitors to the office, how would they apply to others? (This is certainly the group of patients primary care physicians are interested in, but might seem restrictive to a community-oriented epidemiologist.) If these comparisons of physician and patient characteristics are made with the overall populations, if the sampling techniques are clearly described, and if the inclusions and exclusions are defined, the extent of generalizability can be considered. Since these physicians were also involved in the development of the project, they were probably more consistent in interpreting the definitions and better at recording data than is often the case, which should be taken into account when assessing the merits of the study. The report was written, describing in detail what was done and how it was done, and it was left to the reader to decide how to generalize and apply the findings.

Choosing an Appropriate Design

The development of an appropriate design is essential to the successful achievement of the objectives of any research project. Kirkwood (1988) noted that, "No amount of sophisticated analysis can salvage a poorly designed or badly carried out study." The best design for any project is based on several factors: the question being asked, the incidence or prevalence of the condition being studied, whether the investigator has control of any intervention, and whether randomization is appropriate and can be accomplished.

Graziano and Raulin (1989) use the term *level of constraint* to categorize types of research design. Lower levels of constraint allow for wider generalizability, while higher levels allow for more rigorous interpretation of data (for example, imputing causation usually needs a higher level of constraint than does the demonstration of associations). The researcher should choose the design with the highest level of constraint appropriate to the hypothesis and that which is practical, feasible, and ethical in the setting.

Experimental designs have the most constraint, as they are prospective, the intervention is usually controlled by the investigator, and specific inclusions and exclusions are imposed. For controlled clinical trials the interventions should be randomized, and if possible the observers, the treating physicians, and the subjects should all be blind as to treatment group.

Observational studies have less constraint, with decreasing levels of constraint present in cohort, case-control, and cross-sectional studies, respectively. In cohort studies, which are usually prospective in nature, the exposure is not controllable by the investigator: The subjects, some of whom are exposed to the risk factor of interest, are simply followed over time to ascertain the outcomes, and subsequent analysis is done according to exposure status. Case-control designs are retrospective, with sampling carried out according to the disease rather than to the exposure. Identified cases are compared to controls (a group of individuals not having the disease). In cross-sectional designs, data are collected at specified times, without an intervention, and analyzed in relation to the prevalence of factors and the associations between different variables.

Some general principles apply when choosing a design. If the event to be studied is rare, a case-control design is probably necessary. If an intervention exists but cannot be controlled by the investigator (e.g., the development of a positive response to the AIDS virus), then a cohort or case-control design is most appropriate. The test of a new diagnostic tool or therapy requires a randomized, controlled trial in order to achieve the degree of rigor necessary to comfortably recommend a different management approach. However, if disease outcome is imminent death, randomization is usually not ethical and a before/after design may be necessary.

In planning the design, consideration needs to be given to the techniques that will be used to sample the relevant population, to randomly allocate subjects, and to maintain compliance both with the study protocol and with the drug (if one is involved). What will be done with nonresponders or dropouts? All these issues must be resolved before the study begins. Once a particular design has been selected, then the standards related to that design must apply. Detailed discussion of each type of design and their specific standards may be found in most textbooks of epidemiology or statistics (Fletcher, Fletcher, & Wagner, 1982; Sackett, Haynes, & Tugwell, 1985; Hennekens & Buring, 1987; Streiner, Norman, & Blum, 1989).

There are three main types of bias: selection bias, confounding bias, and information bias. Selection bias occurs if the selected subjects differ systematically from those not selected. Confounding bias is likely to exist if the variable of interest is influenced by another variable that is different in the groups being compared. Information bias occurs if there are systematic errors in measurement of one or more of the variables being collected. Bias is most likely to occur in cross-sectional studies and least likely in an experimental trial using a randomized double-blind controlled design. Cohort and case-control studies are intermediate in this potential.

To clarify some of the issues related to appropriate designs for primary care research, examples of studies using four different designs will be presented: experimental trials, cohort studies, case-control studies, and cross-sectional studies. For each design, several major points will be stressed, which might be considered our basic standards for each design.

EXAMPLE: EXPERIMENTAL TRIALS

Does a counseling intervention help people stop smoking? A study by Wilson et al. (1988) was designed to address this question. Seventy community general practices were randomly assigned to three groups. In the group that served as the control, patients who smoked received only usual care. In the "gum-only" group, the physicians agreed to prescribe nicotine gum for their smoking patients; and in the "gum-plus" group, in addition to prescribing the gum, the physicians were trained to give an educational intervention. The self-reported smoking status of all patients was assessed and followed for six months. In some patients the self-reports of smoking were verified by a saliva test. Effectiveness of the gum alone and the gum plus educational intervention was compared to the control group.

In this study, the efficacy of the randomization procedure was checked by comparing the physicians and the patients in each of the three groups. There were no differences in the baseline characteristics of the physicians, while the only difference among the patients was that those who were assigned to the educational intervention group were initially more motivated to stop smoking. Did the motivation of patients influence the outcome?

Double blinding was impossible here, but the participating physicians and patients were not informed of the other interventions, so although they were not blind as to their own involvement, they were as to the contrasting interventions. This is one way to increase the rigor of a study in which the participants cannot be blind.

Some disadvantages of the experimental design in primary care research are that it is often not practical or applicable to the problems of main concern. Conditions of interest may be infrequent, so obtaining a sufficient sample is difficult. The rigor required for the method often eliminates patients whom it would be important to study, such as those with multiple problems, those who are nonattending or noncompliant, or those who for various reasons cannot be managed in an ideal way.

EXAMPLE: COHORT STUDIES

Since 1969 more than 1,400 British general practitioners have been cooperating in a study to ascertain the long-term effects of the birth control pill (Beral, Hannaford, & Kay, 1988; Croft & Hannaford, 1989; Kay & Hannaford, 1988). An initial cohort of 47,000 patients, half on the pill and half not, was recruited over an 18-month period, and has now been followed for more than 20 years. Every six months the physician documents each patient's exposure to the pill as well as any outcomes related to morbidity and mortality. This particular study has made a major contribution to the understanding of the pill's long-term effects.

As demonstrated in this example, the cohort study is very relevant in primary care. It is a powerful method to address many of the problems facing the family physician and is usually the best type of design when exposure to the intervention is not controllable (e.g., infectious diseases, genetic diseases, environmental exposures, and so forth). Cohort studies require that:

- the sample be clearly defined,
- all instances of the exposure be recorded, including duration,
- outcomes be clearly defined and looked for in all individuals, and,
- all subjects be accounted for.

In the British contraceptive study described above, attempts have been made to deal with all of these factors.

There are, however, disadvantages with this design as well. The important outcomes and confounding variables need to be known before the study begins, but this is not always the case, especially with respect to possible confounding variables. For example, in the study described here, 20 years ago the possible association of breast cancer with time of first pregnancy was not known, so the age of first pregnancy was not originally collected and now must be obtained retrospectively (Kay & Hannaford,

1988). At present, it has only been collected in those women who have developed cancer, so appropriate analysis for the effects of this variable is not possible.

Furthermore, in cohort studies, if the time from exposure to disease is long and/or the event rate is low, large samples are necessary and the studies must continue over a long time. Although the British study had more than 400,000 patient-years of data by March 1985, only 18,000 of the original women were still being followed then. And even with this still large number of subjects, many of the subgroups in specific analyses (e.g., breast cancer by age groups) are still small, so tests of significance are not robust. The 95% confidence interval for relative risks in some subgroups still has ranges as large as 0.84 to 55.51 (Kay & Hannaford, 1988).

Another consideration must be the employment of strategies to increase the reliability of the results. These may involve keeping up the interest of the recorders and subjects, maintaining the quality of the data, and ensuring that drop-outs and deaths are recorded accurately. In the British study all these have been accomplished: Regular reports to the participants keep interest high, while original instrument design and constant monitoring help to maintain the integrity of the data. In any long-term project, concise forms are essential: The least amount of recording time possible must be achieved (if regular recording is required, 30 seconds per patient encounter for data collection and recording is probably all that a busy physician will tolerate). Well-designed checkoff cards make this quick, easy, and sufficiently reliable.

EXAMPLE: CASE-CONTROL STUDIES

A family physician noted an association in two of his patients between the reactivation of tuberculosis and the long-term use of nonsteroidal anti-inflammatory agents. This association was reported (Brennan, 1982) and a subsequent case-control study was conducted (Tomasson, Brennan, & Bass, 1984). One hundred and six new and reactivated cases of tuberculosis over a one-year period were identified from the local area, using the Provincial Chest Clinic, pulmonary specialists, and Public Health Department records. The family physicians of these individuals were contacted, and 38 of the cases were matched to another patient in the same physician's practice for age (+/- 3 years), sex, race, and length of time in the practice. There was an equal number of index and control subjects. For each case, the following data were extracted from the patient's medical record: the number of visits to the physician, the number of medications given, and the number of prescriptions for ASA, steroids, and nonsteroidal anti-inflammatory drugs. Comparisons were made between the tuberculosis patients and the control group.

The standards for case-control studies include the following:

- ensuring that all cases (or a random sample) are included,
- defining and selecting an appropriate control sample, and,
- maintaining the integrity and completeness of the data collection.

In primary care few conditions are common. Indeed, most diseases are seen only rarely, and for such entities, it is impractical to do other than case-control studies. In this example, it would have been unethical to do a randomized controlled trial, while a cohort study would have had to be very large and gone on for a long time. A case-control study, in contrast, was both practical and appropriate.

In case-control studies care must be taken in several areas. Were all the cases of tuberculosis found? In this example, cases were derived from different sources to minimize the risk of missing any, but because of lack of information, only about one-third of those found could be followed.

Who are the proper controls? In many case-control studies this is the most crucial design issue. Considerable care must be taken in deciding on the controls, and, if there is a small number of index cases, it may be appropriate to have more than one control case for each: for example, two. Some matching of the cases and controls may be essential, but if matching is too rigid, it may be difficult to find suitable controls, and some information about confounding variables may be lost (e.g., the effects of sex or age).

Case-control studies are by definition retrospective, so all the problems of data collection in retrospective studies are present. Particular attention must be made to ensure accurate and complete data collection.

A British family physician developed the hypothesis that signs and symptoms in respiratory disease were more important than diagnosis in determining treatment with an antibiotic (Howie, 1972). To test this hypothesis, he collected data on the signs and symptoms, diagnoses, and treatment from more than 500 respiratory illness cases from 62 general practices. The hypothesis was supported, and this study led to a number of others that elaborated on the implications of the findings (Howie, 1973, 1974, 1976; Howie & Hutchison, 1978).

In this study, the hypothesis was a general one; the reasons for any differences were not at issue. The simple question permitted simple data collection, such as basic demographics of the reporting physician and the patient variables described above. Although brief and simple, these data were sufficient to test the hypothesis. Because the physicians were self-selected and because of the nature of the data collection (lack of standardization of reporting physicians), it would have been inappropriate to try to interpret the data in more detail. Nonetheless, two things were achieved. First, the data collection methods were feasible and could be accomplished, and some of the difficulties of data collection became apparent. Second, valuable data were obtained which enabled further hypothesis development.

Larger and more extensive cross-sectional studies than this one have been done: For example, much of the knowledge of the symptoms and psychological concomitants of the menopause has been accumulated through such studies in several countries, and most vital statistics databases are derived from repeated cross-sectional surveys.

Ensuring the Objectivity of Measures

Several steps must be taken to ensure the objectivity and the appropriateness of the data collected. These are discussed in detail below.

First, all diagnoses involved in a study must be clearly defined, and inclusions and exclusions must be elaborated. The investigators and their assistants must be able to decide whether any potential subject has the disease or condition and meets the inclusion and exclusion criteria. These decisions must be consistent across all study personnel involved in entering subjects into the study, administering the instruments, and/or collecting data. One of the hallmarks of a good multicenter or multipractice trial is the successful effort to minimize differences between subjects from different centers. This is best accomplished through initially having an agreed-upon protocol for screening and entering potential subjects. Ideally, personnel from each center will help develop and/or approve of that protocol and, as the study progresses, should hold regular meetings to discuss it, along with issues of recruitment or any other problems that may arise.

The data collection instruments for the proposed study must be reliable and valid. If previously developed instruments are being used, their characteristics should be considered to see if they are acceptable; if new instruments are created, they must be tested for their reliability and validity before the study is undertaken. (Some testing of instruments can be done during the course of the study, but if results are unacceptable, then the study is in serious trouble.) When several instruments measuring the same construct are available, the most objective one should be used (e.g., a company work record rather than a self-report of work history). When choosing the instruments to be used to make the subsequent analysis more powerful, the researcher should review the type of variables to be collected, the type of statistical analysis, and the availability of subjects.

As mentioned above, standardization of observers is essential, especially when there is more than one. If there is any subjective element in the use of an instrument, observers need to be trained both to apply the instruments and to standardize their responses and interpretations. At some point during the project, intra- and inter-observer variation must be measured. Whenever appropriate, all possible efforts should be made to keep investigators, data handlers, and subjects blind as to the experimental manipulations. This is not always feasible, however; for example, if there are side-effects to a medication, either observers or subjects may guess (more often than not correctly) whether they are receiving a placebo or the active ingredient.

EXAMPLE

A family physician is coordinating a randomized, double-blind, controlled trial, comparing drugs A and B in treating hypertension in the elderly. Control of blood pressure and quality of life will be contrasted between the two groups. Because of the need for more than 100 subjects in each group, the study is being done in eight different sites, each entering about 25 patients. Patients with diabetes, asthma, cardiovascular disease, or prior congestive heart failure are to be excluded. What efforts should be made to ensure that this study is done appropriately?

Questions to be asked here include: What are the criteria for the diagnoses of hypertension, diabetes, cardiovascular disease, and congestive heart failure? For example, is hypertension defined as an elevation of diastolic pressure, of systolic pressure, or both, and what levels constitute hypertension in this study? Do all the participating physicians understand and agree to each of the criteria for inclusion and exclusion, and will these criteria be interpreted in the same way by all? Ideally, the physicians should meet as a group to reach a consensus on these factors.

The blood pressure readings must be objective, so calibration of the instruments being used to measure blood pressure must be carried out. The observers must be trained to all take the blood pressure in the same way: for example, sitting, taken in both arms, using the same cut-off point, and after the same period of rest. Ideally, a machine that randomly changes the zero point before the blood pressure is taken (a "random zero sphygmomanometer") could be used to minimize the rounding bias. (The value of the blood pressure is corrected after the reading is taken.)

Other considerations include the following. What is to be used to measure quality of life? Does a valid, reliable, disease-specific instrument exist, and was it developed and tested on a population similar to the one under study? Drugs A and B must be manufactured in a form that looks, tastes, and seems the same to both the subjects and the physicians. Constant effort should be made to keep records on all subjects entered into the study. Drop-outs must be noted, noncompliance assessed, and all relevant outcomes recorded. As much as possible, no subjects should be lost to follow-up, even if they do not complete the study. All these areas need to be addressed and possible inconsistencies between the different settings resolved.

Drawing Justified Interpretations

When a study is complete, several principles must be kept in mind as the results are interpreted and disseminated: (1) all subjects must be accounted for, (2) appropriate statistics must be used, (3) interpretation of the data should be appropriate and clinical significance addressed, and (4) the consistency of the results with other studies should be considered.

In analytic studies it is not valid to first collect the data, look at the results of a preliminary descriptive analysis, and then decide on the statistical analyses. The specific statistical procedure to be used depends on the type of study, the format of the variables, and whether differences or associations are to be tested. These should all be in place at the beginning of the study. If the investigators are not familiar with the requirements for statistical analysis, consultation is necessary.

All subjects initially considered for the study should be accounted for, including those excluded after the study began, drop-outs, and those lost to follow-up. In the final report it is useful to include a table presenting this data (the number of subjects in each category and demographic data on them by category). This information will help a reader decide if there are biases in the results because of the loss of subjects.

Over-interpretation of the data must be guarded against. First and foremost, demonstration of association is not a proof of causality: Specific designs and analyses are required to impute causality. Even when associations are demonstrated, all possible confounding variables must be considered and discussed. Statistically significant findings are not necessarily clinically significant: For example, if the number of subjects is large, statistical significance is often easy to demonstrate. A true difference of 2 mm of Hg blood pressure between patients on drug A versus drug B is probably clinically unimportant. The cost, side-effects, and ease of use of the drugs may be more important in choosing a therapy than a minimal difference in blood pressure reading.

If the study showed no difference between the study and the control groups, power calculations must be done: That is, the beta error (the probability of getting, by chance, a negative result when in fact there is a difference) must be calculated. If it is high, then only tentative conclusions should be drawn. In many instances, presenting the data and the confidence limits around them gives the reader a better understanding of the significance of the results. Last but not least, interpretation of the results should not be generalized to a population other than one similar to the one from which the sample came.

New and innovative discoveries in primary care are exciting. Nonetheless, cautious interpretation is prudent when the results of a study are counterintuitive or are inconsistent with previous findings. Conversely, if the results are similar to those obtained in different circumstances or in different populations, confidence in their reliability increases.

EXAMPLE

Consider a hypothetical example. A study has shown that for healthy, asymptomatic North American males between the ages of 40 and 65 with cholesterol levels above 240, there is a 10% lowering of cardiovascular mortality and a 15% lowering of cardiac morbidity after seven years for those who are treated with a specific cholesterol-lowering agent. These findings are comparable to those of several similar studies of other cholesterol-lowering agents.

Only one main conclusion from this study would be valid: That there is an association between the taking of the drug and changes in cardiovascular mortality and morbidity in this population. Because other studies have yielded similar results, this conclusion is more strongly supported. As yet, however, causation is not demonstrated, nor can these findings be extrapolated to other ethnic groups, to the female population, or to symptomatic patients. In this study there was no statistically significant difference in *total* mortality between the drug-treated group and the control group: Given this, are the differences in cardiovascular outcomes clinically significant? Are there confounding variables, and if so, what is the magnitude of their effects? Although this study adds to the accumulated knowledge in the field, by itself it is probably not enough to be used to make major recommendations for changes in patient management. Interpreted with other, similar studies, it can be used either to point to further areas for research or to suggest specific changes in management.

Conclusion

Rigorous analytic research in primary care is possible. It requires both understanding and maintaining the standards that are appropriate to the study being undertaken. At present, researchers must follow, to the best extent possible, the standards that exist for scientific research in related fields. However, they should continue to formulate and develop specific standards for primary care research, either by adaptation of existing standards or by creation of new ones. The time has come when the scientific community can expect primary care research to be based on criteria as rigorous as those for any other research discipline.

References

Beral, V., Hannaford, P., & Kay. C. (1988). Oral contraceptive use and malignancies of the genital tract. Results from the Royal College of General Practitioners' oral contraception study. *Lancet, 2,* 1331-1335.

Brennan, M. (1982). Latent tuberculosis and anti-inflammatory agents. *Canadian Medical Association Journal, 126,* 21.

Croft, P., & Hannaford, P. C. (1989). Risk factors for acute myocardial infarction in women: Evidence from the Royal College of General Practitioners' oral contraception study. *British Medical Journal, 298,* 165-168.

Feinstein, A. R. (1989). *Intellectual crisis in clinical medicine.* Keynote address presented at the annual meeting of the North American Primary Care Research Group, San Antonio, Texas.

Fletcher, R. H., Fletcher, S. W., & Wagner, E. H. (1982). *Clinical epidemiology: The essentials.* Baltimore: Williams and Wilkins.

Graziano, A. M., & Raulin, M. L. (1989). *Research methods: A process of inquiry.* New York: Harper & Row.

Headache Study Group of The University of Western Ontario, The. (1986). Predictors of outcome in headache patients presenting to family physicians: A one-year prospective study. *Headache, 26,* 285-294.

Hennekens, C. H., & Buring, J. E. (1987). *Epidemiology in medicine.* Boston: Little, Brown.

Howie, J. G. (1972). Diagnosis: The Achilles heel. *Journal of the Royal College of General Practice, 22,* 310-315.

Howie, J.G . (1973). A new look at respiratory illness in general practice: A reclassification of respiratory illness based on antibiotic prescribing. *Journal of the Royal College of General Practice, 23,* 895-904.

Howie, J. G. (1974). Further observations on diagnosis and management of general practice respiratory illness using simulated patient consultations. *British Medical Journal, 2,* 540-543.

Howie, J. G. (1976). Clinical judgement and antibiotic use in general practice. *British Medical Journal, 2,* 1061-1064.

Howie, J. G., & Hutchison, K. R. (1978). Antibiotics and respiratory illness in general practice: Prescribing policy and workload. *British Medical Journal, 2,* 1342.

Kay, C., & Hannaford, P. C. (1988). Breast cancer and the pill: A further report from the Royal College of General Practitioners' oral contraception study. *British Journal of Cancer, 58* (5), 675-680.

Kirkwood, B. K. (1988). *Essentials of medical statistics.* London: Blackwell Scientific Publications.

Sackett, D. L., Haynes, R. B., & Tugwell, P. (1985). *Clinical epidemiology: A basic science for clinical medicine.* Toronto: Little, Brown.

Streiner, D. L., Norman, G. R., & Blum, H. M. (1989). *Epidemiology.* Toronto: B. C. Decker.

Tomasson, H. O., Brennan, M., & Bass, M. J. (1984). Tuberculosis and nonsteroidal anti-inflammatory drugs. *Canadian Medical Association Journal, 130* (3), 275-278.

Wilson, D. M., Taylor, D. W., Gilbert, J. R., Best, J. A., Lindsay, E. A., Willms, D. G., & Singer, J. (1988). A randomized trial of a family physician intervention for smoking cessation. *Journal of the American Medical Association, 260* (11), 1570-1574.

7 Case Reports—Boon or Bane?

BRIAN A. P. MORRIS

This chapter discusses the form of medical communication called the case report. To open, I will share what some eminent medical writers have said about case reports.

David Sackett and his colleagues (1985, p. 229) have described them as "methodologically weak" and "prone to interpretation." An editorialist (Soffer, 1976) in the *Archive of Internal Medicine,* described them as "the most abused and misunderstood form of medical communication." In the *Canadian Medical Association Journal (CMAJ),* Peter Morgan (1985) wrote that "the collection of case reports that trails after the editorials, letters, reviews, and scientific studies is probably the least distinguished section of a general medical journal . . . generally no more than enhanced anecdotes." And one final comment, "this genre . . . has been widely abused, its quality [is] mediocre" (DeBakey & Debakey, 1983).

As I consider those descriptions, I wonder what I'm doing writing this chapter. Possibly the answer lies in what some other eminent experts have said. William Osler (Debakey & Debakey, 1983) is said to have enjoined his students to "communicate or publish short notes on *anything* that is striking or new." Case reports have more recently been called "a rich source of information" (Debakey & Debakey, 1983), "valuable tools that have led to many medical advances" (Coccia & Ausman, 1987), and "a valuable teaching exercise" (Soffer, 1976).

So, with these positive words in mind, my discussion continues. The entity that I will examine here is called a *case report* if it involves just one (or occasionally two) subjects, and a *case series* if it involves more. Medical journals include greater or fewer numbers of these types of articles, depending on the prestige, audience, and style of the publication. For instance, in 1988 the *Canadian Family Physician* published just five case reports, while the CMAJ published 41 out of a grand total of 177 scientific articles, representing 23% of their total. Some of the topics covered by case reports in CMAJ included "Three Cases of Diflunisal Hypersensitivity," "Fatal Reaction to Peanut Antigen in Almond Icing," "Renal Revascularization for Acute Anuria," and so on. (There was also one that could only have been published in Canada: "Laceration of the Common Peroneal Nerve by a Skate Blade"!) I think the fact that case studies represent such a high proportion of articles in journals such as the CMAJ behooves medical writers to study this genre. If it is going to be done, let us do it well.

To illustrate the potential importance of case studies, I will present a selection of reports that have been crucial in introducing new diseases or generating hypotheses that have led to medical breakthroughs.

The first example is a report that was published in *Arthritis and Rheumatism* in 1976 (Steer, Malaivista, Snydman, & Andiman, 1976), describing a cluster of arthritis in children and adults in a small town in Connecticut. Most of these 35 patients developed a sudden onset of pain and swelling in a knee, often accompanied by low-grade fever, severe myalgias, and maculopapular rashes. Specific tests for a number of rheumatological diseases and viruses were negative, and the authors suggested that this outbreak of arthritis in the small town of Lyme might be "a new clinical entity." To claim in a case report that a syndrome described represents a new clinical entity is indeed a courageous act; one that, it has been suggested "ought usually to be eschewed and that distinction [be] not conferred by oneself but by posterity" (Huth, 1982, pp. 58-63).

An important benefit of a good case study is that it can stimulate, either directly or indirectly, further definitive quantitative studies. This is illustrated by my second example: the story of what is now called Toxic Shock Syndrome. The first record I could find of this syndrome, called by this name, was in a 1978 *Lancet* article (Todd, Fishaut, Kapral, & Welch, 1978), titled "Toxic Shock

Syndrome Associated with Phage-Group-1 Staphylococci." This report described seven children, ages eight to 17 years, who presented with what we now recognize as the defining symptoms and signs of Toxic Shock Syndrome. The authors described the steps they took to exclude other known childhood infections and noted that the causative bacterium was isolated from various mucosal sites, including the vagina. But at no point did they make any mention of menstrual status or even the sex of these children, although the one case that they described in detail was indeed a 15-year-old girl. In their discussion, the authors admitted to their perplexity as to why Toxic Shock Syndrome affected older children rather than younger ones, who are affected by so many other exanthems.

This case report, although it lacked some vital pieces of information, nonetheless raised questions. Subsequent case reports described the syndrome as happening in young adults, detailed the fact that 95% of those affected were women, and established the association with menses. All of this provided the groundwork for a major quantitative study. It was almost exactly two years later that the *New England Journal of Medicine* reported a case control study involving 52 cases and 52 age- and sex-matched controls that proved the association between tampon use and toxic shock (Shands et al., 1980). Again we see the sequence: a case report that is stimulating, thought-provoking, and leads, in fairly short order, to definitive answers being obtained.

One more example I hope will be sufficient. *The American Journal of Dermatopathology* might not seem a very likely publication in which the most important new disease of the century should be heralded, but so it was. In the summer of 1981, Gottlieb et al. published a case report that was the very model of brevity: just 50 lines of single-column print, five references, and half a dozen figures. The title said it all: "A Preliminary Communication on Extensively Disseminated Kaposi's Sarcoma in Young Homosexual Men." This was the first report of anything that you and I would now call AIDS. Again, as in all good case reports, questions were raised. For instance, "this sudden, very high incidence of the condition in male homosexuals suggests an epidemic and raises the possibility of an infectious cause." Then, in a masterstroke of prescience, the authors predicted that this disease "threatens to become rampant in homosexuals."

Another case study was published just a few weeks later in a rather better-known medical journal, *Lancet*, and described a series of eight cases of Kaposi's sarcoma in homosexual men (Hymes et al., 1981). This report, too, hinted at the possibility of a sexually transmitted disease, and also discussed various "observations supporting immunosuppression as the underlying factor."

This particular saga unfolded very quickly. On December 10, 1981, *The New England Journal of Medicine* published a lead article, titled "Pneumocystis Carinii Pneumonia and Mucosal Candidiasis in Previously Healthy Homosexual Men" (Gotlieb et al., 1981). One of these men also had Kaposi's sarcoma, and I find it fascinating that just three months after the original reports, it was already well known that pneumocystis carinii pneumonia and Kaposi's sarcoma traveled together in male homosexuals.

And so you have it: AIDS first described in a humble case report in a subspecialist journal.

I hope the above examples have illustrated the occasionally dramatic importance of case reports. They represent a qualitative method of study, and to be done well they should involve a qualitative difference in our concepts of disease processes. Good case studies must at least suggest a qualitative jump in knowledge; at their best, they make a quantum leap. At their worst, case reports creep by millimeters: I refer to the unfortunate habit of submitting "me, too" reports—such as one of my early published efforts, "Erythema Multiforme Major Following Use of Diclofenac" (Morris & Remtulla, 1985). Erythema multiforme major, or Stevens-Johnson Syndrome, had already been reported following the use of half a dozen other nonsteroidal anti-inflammatories, so we should not have been surprised that it happened following the use of this drug, even though it had not specifically been reported. Nonetheless, a colleague and I saw fit to write it up, and the CMAJ saw fit to publish it.

I will summarize the types of cases that *are* worth reporting (Huth, 1982). First, of course, is the unique case, such as the report on Lyme disease. Discovery, description, and publication of a truly unique case is more than just a professional triumph for the clinician involved: It can be important for medicine as a whole. In deciding whether a set of disease manifestations is indeed new, however, the clinician needs to rely on more than memory and must carefully search the literature. Medical terminology changes, as do investigative techniques, so some work is required to ensure that a case is in fact unique.

The second type of case that often warrants publication is that of unexpected association, as in the association of two very rare illnesses such as Kaposi's sarcoma and pneumocystis carinii pneumonia. Two diseases or syndromes found in one patient may suggest a causal relationship, or it may just be coincidence. Being able to suggest a link, as in the suggestions of viral etiology and immunosuppression, certainly strengthens the argument and allows further studies to be aimed specifically at establishing or disproving causation.

The final type of case worthy of discussion is that of unexpected events, such as a truly unexpected and important side effect of a drug, or an unexpected recovery from a disease previously thought to be fatal. Again, if causal association is to be believed, it should at least be supported by exclusion of alternative explanations.

Which types of case reports should you and I *avoid*? I've already offered an example of the "me, too" report, which I've named after a habit my two daughters have. If one daughter comes in, saying that she saw a fire engine on the way home from school, the other will of course pipe up "me, too." Too many medical authors succumb to the same temptation: "I've seen this!" "Me, too!"

Another type of report to be avoided is the numerical one-upmanship report, which says that if Smith reported the successful removal of a 226-pound ovarian mass last year, then the 227-pound ovarian mass that I removed yesterday should be reported. The extra pound does not increase medical knowledge in any way and does not warrant publication.

Also, avoid the temptation to write up a case in which you, the author, just got lucky and stumbled onto a diagnosis. And finally, shun the case report that describes a disease so incredibly rare that none of us will ever see it, but nonetheless we are always urged to "keep it in the back of your mind." (The back of my mind is so full of these little titbits that I sometimes have trouble getting my head off the pillow in the morning.)

Let us now look at how a case report evolves and should be written. Several good style guides are listed in the references

(Debakey & Debakey, 1983; Huth, 1982); here, I will just offer a brief overview.

If you believe that a patient under your care is indeed showing a new constellation of signs and symptoms or is exhibiting a side effect that hasn't been reported before, or you've discovered a new cure for this ailment: The first step is to check it out. Ask colleagues, check the texts. A careful literature search, with or without the help of a computer, needs to be not just done but documented. If you go on to write up the case report, a statement such as "a Medline English-language search was done, using the following key words for the following period of time" is both convincing and useful to editors and readers. And, however sad this makes you, you may indeed find out that your case is not unique. However, in this situation, nothing is lost but your excitement and anticipation—and much better to find out now than to have an editor point it out to you after you've submitted a finished work.

You will have already, it is hoped, carefully documented the case itself. This may involve getting additional laboratory information, to exclude other possible diagnoses that you've come up with in your literature search, or other necessary data. Finally, after all this is done, the thoughtful clinician steps back a pace or two and decides whether the case warrants reporting. Would its publication be just another item on a CV, or will it in any important way advance medical knowledge? If you, the author, saw this case reported in a general medical journal, would you stop to read it and marvel at it, or would you pass it over?

If you decide to write up the report, many journals offer very clear instructions in their "Guidelines to Authors" with regard to format, length, number of references, number of illustrations, and so on. One style guide (Debakey & Debakey, 1983) recommends constant consideration of the ABCs of writing case reports—the initials standing for Accuracy, Brevity, and Conciseness. If a report is to be fewer than 1,000 words, every one of those words must be important.

The format is quite standard. Start with an introduction that describes in just a couple of sentences what there is about your case that justifies the report; that is, why you feel the situation is unique or unexpected. Follow this with the description: an account of the case in narrative form, including only those positive and negative findings that are important in diagnosis, and only those elements of the patient's course that are crucial to understanding its uniqueness.

The discussion, also called the commentary or conclusion, is the real argument of the case report. To be fair and considerate, present both the evidence in favor of your argument and whatever shortfalls or weaknesses you feels are present. Contradictory evidence must be fully and fairly presented. This is also the place for unanswered questions, which, if the case report is serving its role properly, will stimulate other researchers to construct the appropriate studies to prove etiology or otherwise complete the knowledge suggested here.

I hope these guidelines clarify the differences between a case report and a case study. The case *report* has two important attributes: conciseness of style and some element of uniqueness in subject matter. A case *study*, while it usually has the second of these, does not require the first: It can be as lengthy as a chapter or even a book, since it requires an in-depth, exhaustive description of the case in hand, as well as some conclusion or new interpretation based on it.

In closing, I would like to offer a philosophical look. Some of the other research tools described in this volume look at populations or averages: the medical equivalent of studying a forest by flying over it at 5,000 feet. How very different it is to walk through that forest and look at one tree, whether it be the tallest or the shortest, and examine it in detail, studying the structure of a single leaf, feeling the texture of the bark, examining the tiny crevices in the surface in which a microcosm can dwell. When looking at populations or forests, the extremes are lumped in with the medians and the modes. Can we not learn something from the outliers? From the oddities? From the unusual cases that stimulate new hypotheses? I think the answer is yes.

References

Coccia, C. T., & Ausman, J. I. (1987). Is a case report an anecdote? *Surgical Neurology, 28,* 111-113.

DeBakey, L., & DeBakey, S. (1983). The case report. I. Guidelines for preparation. *International Journal of Cardiology, 4,* 357-364.

Gottlieb, M. S., Schroff, R., Schanker, H. M., Weisman, J. D., Fan, P. T., Wolf, R. A., & Saxon, A. (1981). Pneumocystis carinii pneumonia and mucosal candidiasis in previously healthy homosexual men. *New England Journal of Medicine, 305,* 1425-1431.

Gottlieb, G. J., Ragaz, A., Vogel, J. V., Friedman-Kien, A., Rywiln, A. M., Weiner, E. A., & Ackerman, A. B. (1981). A preliminary communication on extensively disseminated Kaposi's sarcoma in young homosexual men. *American Journal of Dematopathology, 3*(2), 111-114.

Huth, E. J. (1982). *How to write and publish papers in the medical sciences.* Philadelphia: ISI Press.

Hymes, K. B., Greene, J. B., Marcus, A., William, D. C., Cheung, T., Prose, N. S., Ballard, H., & Laubenstein, L. J. (1981). Kaposi's sarcoma in homosexual men—a report of eight cases. *Lancet, 2,* 598-600.

Morgan, P. P. (1985). Why case reports. *Canadian Medical Association Journal, 133,* 353.

Morris, B. A. & Remtulla, S. S. (1985). Erythema multiforme major following use of diclofenac. *Canadian Medical Association Journal, 133*(7), 665.

Sackett, D. L., Haynes, R. B., & Tugwell, P. (1985). *Clinical epidemiology.* Toronto: Little, Brown.

Shands, K. N., Schmid, G. P., Dan, B. B., Blum, D., Guidotti, R. J., Hargrett, N. T., Anderson, R. L., Hill, D. L., Broomr, C. V., Band, J. D., & Fraser, D. W. (1980). Toxic-shock syndrome in menstruating women. *New England Journal of Medicine, 303,* 1436-1442.

Soffer, A. (1976). Case reports in the Archives of Internal Medicine. *Archives of Internal Medicine, 136,* 1090.

Steer, A. C., Malaivista, S. E., Snydman, D. R., & Andiman, W. A. (1976). A cluster of arthritis in children and adults in Lyme, Connecticut. *Arthritis and Rheumatology, 19*(4), 824. (Abstract).

Todd, J., Fishaut, M., Kapral, F., & Welch, T. (1978). Toxic-shock syndrome associated with phage-group-I staphylococci. *Lancet, 2,* 1116-1118.

8 Research in Primary Care: The Qualitative Approach

CECIL G. HELMAN

Introduction

The main concerns of primary care are the mental and physical health of individuals, usually within the context of their families, as well as the health of the family itself, seen as a unit or as a small community of individuals. For both of these tasks, research, as well as diagnosis and treatment, has to move beyond the limited agenda set by other branches of medicine. Its emphasis has to shift—and indeed has already begun to—in the direction of being an applied social science as well as an applied medical science.

To be an applied social scientist, however, the physician requires a knowledge of some of the key concepts of social science and the research methodologies based on those concepts. In this chapter I will discuss one of the oldest of the social sciences, cultural (or social) anthropology, and why it is particularly relevant to primary care research.

Anthropology, the study of human beings, has been called "the most scientific of the humanities, and the most humane of the sciences" ("More anthropology," 1980). Its aim is the holistic study of our species, including its origins, social and political organization, religions, rituals, languages, customs, and worldviews. A new branch of anthropology, medical anthropology, concerns itself with how people in different cultures and social groups explain the causes of ill health, the types of treatment they believe in, and to whom they turn if they do get ill. It is also the study of how these beliefs and behaviors relate to biological and psychological changes in the human organism, in both health and disease (Helman, 1984a).

In the modern Western world, especially in urban areas, the primary care or family physician is likely to encounter an increasingly diverse patient population (Like & Steiner, 1986). This population now often includes immigrants, refugees, emigrés, and guestworkers, as well as foreign tourists, students, and businesspeople. There are also the members of indigenous populations, such as Native Americans and Native Canadians, and the followers of different cults, lifestyles, and religions. Furthermore, the physician may be separated from his or her patients by barriers of social class, gender, color, or education (Helman, 1987). To provide more humane, efficient, and culturally appropriate primary care to this diverse population, new modalities of research must be developed, especially those with a more qualitative approach.

In this chapter I propose to examine four key questions in relation to primary care research:

- What are the key concepts underlying medical anthropology and its qualitative methods of research? What do we mean by "qualitative" research methods, and how do they differ from other approaches to medical research?
- What are the strengths and weaknesses of both qualitative and quantitative research methods?
- What are the sorts of problems in primary care that can best be examined by a more qualitative approach?
- What types of clinically relevant research projects can be realistically carried out in a primary care setting, using qualitative methodology?

Medical Anthropology: Some Basic Concepts

In understanding human behavior, anthropologists have developed the concept of culture. This can be understood as an inherited "lens" of shared concepts and rules of meaning through which the members of a group or society perceive the world they live in, and which guides their daily behavior in relation to other people, to the natural environment, and to supernatural forces or gods. Culture is a set of guidelines, both implicit and explicit, which every individual inherits as a member of a particular society. It is transmitted from generation to generation by the use of language, symbols, and rituals, and without it neither the cohesion nor the continuity of any human group would be possible.

Hall (1983) has called the deepest, most inaccessible level of culture "primary level culture," and proposes that this provides the "hidden cultural grammar" of our lives. This set of unconscious assumptions and rules of behavior controls much of human activity, but individuals are rarely aware of it, or of the possibility of a clash between incompatible and hidden cultural grammars. There are also more accessible levels of culture, such as rituals, customs, and festivals. This visible level is more amenable to change than culture at the primary level.

Within a culture there are subcultures, which are smaller groups of people who, while sharing many aspects of the larger culture, also have unique, distinctive features of their own. Subcultures include religious, ethnic, and social minorities; institutions such as hospitals, clubs, and universities; the followers of certain religions or lifestyles; and certain professional groups (such as the medical profession, which has developed its own distinctive worldview, social organization, language, and rituals). In addition, to some extent in some societies, men and women have different though parallel "cultures," while each family has its own small subculture. A culture clash can occur between members of different cultures or subcultures; one place that has the potential for such a clash is the doctor-patient relationship.

Although culture is a useful concept, it can be misunderstood or misused (Helman, 1990). Cultures are never static, homogeneous or isolated, nor are they the preserve only of the poor and the powerless. One should also always avoid using cultural stereotypes or using culture as an excuse for "victim-blaming," since culture may be a misleading explanation for health inequalities in society (Mares, Henley & Baxter, 1985). Low incomes, unemployment, poor diet, substandard housing, limited educational opportunities, crime, and religious or ethnic discrimination may all relate to the origin, perpetuation, recognition, and treatment of ill health. Culture alone, therefore, is only a partial explanation for behavior, since one must include subculture, education, socioeconomic status, and personal factors such as age, personality, experience, gender, and appearance.

The sum of these influences, many of which are hidden from the primary care physician, have important influences on many aspects of people's lives, including their beliefs, behaviors, perceptions, language, religion, family structure, residential patterns, gender roles, child-rearing practices, diet, dress, body image, explanations for ill health, self-medication, compliance with medical treatment, and concepts of time and space (Foster & Anderson, 1978; Hall, 1969; Harwood, 1981). Such beliefs and behaviors may be either protective of health or pathogenic, depending on the context (Helman, 1984a; Landy, 1977). For example, the practice of endogamy, whereby individuals must marry kinsfolk from their own family, clan, or tribe, may lead over time to the "pooling" of recessive genes, with an increased incidence of inherited disorders such as hemophilia, thalassemia major, Tay Sachs disease, and sickle cell anemia. A culture that promotes risk-taking and competitive behavior among males, or increased consumption of alcohol and tobacco, may also be regarded as pathogenic to some individuals within that culture. Lay health beliefs about HIV infection and AIDS can influence sexual behavior and consequent levels of risk (Warwick, Aggleton, & Homand, 1988). Several generations of a family choosing to live under one roof may be protective of health in some ways, such as providing mutual support, additional income and resources, and sharing of household tasks and child care; but such a pattern may also be dangerous in the presence of an infectious disease, such as tuberculosis.

A further concept in medical anthropology is the distinction between disease and illness (Helman, 1981; Kleinman, Eisenberg & Good, 1978). "Disease" is the biomedical view of ill health based on the scientific paradigm: It emphasizes mind-body dualism and the reduction of ill health to observable and quantifiable abnormalities in the structure or function of the human body. It usually involves decontextualization of the patient, from his social, cultural, or religious background, his worldview, hopes, and fears. Diseases are seen as entities that are universal in form, content, and treatment, whatever the sociocultural context in which they appear. "Illness" refers to the patient's subjective response to being unwell; how he and those around him perceive the origin, significance, impact and prognosis of this event; how it affects his daily life and behavior or relationships with others; and the steps he takes to remedy the situation. As Cassell (1978) remarked, illness is "what the patient feels when he goes to the doctor," while disease is "what he has on the way home from the doctor's office."

In most cases, illness and disease coexist, but one may have illness (a general feeling of being unwell, tired, or unhappy) without a physiological disease, or a disease (e.g., asymptomatic hypertension, carcinoma-in-situ, or HIV infection) without an illness. The same disease in different cultural groups, families, or individuals may have different meanings and thus cause different "illnesses."

A final concept relevant to qualitative research is the role of context in doctor-patient communication (Helman, 1984b). Hall (1977) suggests two types of communication: "low context," where the majority of the message is vested in the explicit code of communication (e.g., the information carried on a computer screen or on an X-ray plate), and "high context," where most of the information is carried either by the physical environment in which the communication takes place (such as a doctor's office, hospital ward, outpatient clinic, or the patient's home) or by the internalized prior experience, expectations, attitudes, and culture of the two parties involved. Much of the communication in primary care is "high context," with doctor-patient communication being influenced by these hidden, invisible dimensions of "external context" and "internal context," which develop over time and can be discovered only by a more ethnographic approach to research.

Ethnographic Research: Methods and Concepts

As anthropology was mostly developed in nonliterate societies (where questionnaires, written answers, laboratory experiments, and psychometric testing were not applicable or were difficult to carry out), it has developed its own specific research methodology, known as ethnography or fieldwork (Crane & Angrosino, 1974). This involves "participant observation," usually in small-scale societies, where the researcher lives for a lengthy period in order to understand the people's way of life and how they make sense of the world they live in. He observes their behavior, customs, rituals, religion, social organization, economy, and relationship with the environment, and compares this with the explanations that members of the group share about how and why they live as they do. A second stage is the comparative approach, which seeks to distill the key features of each society and compare it with similar cultures, in order to draw general conclusions about the universal nature of human beings and their social groupings.

In the ethnography of a group of people, there are three levels of phenomena that must be examined:

1. what the ethnographer observes that people actually do;
2. what these people say they think, believe, or do; and
3. what these people actually think or believe.

Level 1 data are gathered by the use of ethnographic fieldwork and participant observation, and level 2 data from interviews, questionnaires, recorded statements, or written materials. Level 3 can be inferred only from the observed data from level 1, and includes phenomena at the level of the personal unconscious, as well as "primary level culture." For example, a physician may warn his patients of the dangers of smoking, yet smoke himself. One can infer here a hidden belief system underlying his behavior: for example, of being lucky or resistant to bronchial carcinoma, or even of being deserving of such a condition. Anthropologists have often reported such discrepancies among these three levels, particularly between stated beliefs and observed actions, and this highlights the value of ethnography as a supplementary technique.

The anthropological approach, as Keesing (1981) points out, is "concerned with meanings rather than measurements, with the texture of everyday life in communities rather than formal abstractions." Anthropologists have "fallen back on human powers to learn, understand and communicate" and "avoided many of the devices that spuriously objectify human encounters," especially in trying to understand such phenomena as myths, rituals, worldviews, and the meanings given to everyday life. Peacock

(1986) describes the "interpretive" viewpoint in anthropology that "no facts exist independent of perceivers . . . 'fact' is seen as a construction reflecting both the perspective of perceivers and the world that they perceive." He recognizes, therefore, that the presence of the researcher may influence the phenomena under study. To some extent, this perspective resembles Tolstoy's remark (1930) about art as "the interpretation of the environment through the medium of a temperament." However, as Kleinman (1983) points out, qualitative ethnography is *not* purely a subjective approach; it is a well developed and systematic method of enquiry involving highly trained investigators, and it usually also includes the collection of quantitative data, such as measures of health (height, weight, disease, and malnutrition incidence), diet, caloric intake, population census, land use, crop output, migration and residential patterns, genealogies, allocation of resources, and certain forms of psychological testing. Anthropological research usually includes, therefore, a mixture of quantitative and qualitative approaches, of positivist as well as interpretive viewpoints.

The systematic procedures of fieldwork (Crane & Angrosino, 1974) ensure considerable agreement and repeatability among different researchers working among the same group of people. However, anthropology recognizes that both the personal attributes of the investigator (e.g., age, gender, experience, ethnic background) and the techniques of enquiry (collection of life histories, narratives, worldviews, genealogies, myths, legends, rituals, and the meanings given to daily life) may influence the phenomena under investigation.

Anthropological techniques also include the use of openended or semistructured interviews, either tape-recorded or conducted with questionnaires. The emphasis on questionnaires that have some open-ended component not only avoids reducing complex human phenomena to the "thin" slice (i.e., "low context" data) gathered by a limited number of questions, but also allows space for what Peacock (1986) terms the "unanticipated realities of field work," whereby "one may enter the field with a specific question or hypothesis, but in the field one encounters something challenging the very formulation of that question; one realizes that the question is misleading or irrelevant." Furthermore, such an approach, which is similar to the "free-association" technique of psychoanalysis, may allow a "thicker" (more "high context") slice of human experience and meanings to emerge.

The qualitative approach can be contrasted with the positivist, more quantitative approach of most medical research. This is based on the logical structure of scientific empiricism, with the emphasis on data that can be tested and verified by repeatable experiments (Kaplan, 1968). It begins with a hypothesis, which is then tested by systematic investigation, and the data thus generated either confirm or invalidate the hypothesis. Like the disease perspective, this emphasizes numerical data and statistics, and research is usually carried out on larger patient populations.

Comparison of Quantitative and Qualitative Approaches

Both qualitative and quantitative research methods have their own strengths and weaknesses.

The positivist, quantitative approach produces data that is objectively verifiable, and repeatable by systematic experiment. It is able to quantify and statistically analyze data, which are thus precisely defined. Its emphasis in medical research on "low context" physiological data (e.g., levels of particular blood cells, hormones, or enzymes) universalizes the study of all those whose bodies contain these cells or substances, but it excludes such phenomena as context, meaning, worldview, religion, beliefs, and behaviors, all of which are also relevant to mental or physical health. The use of diagnostic technology, both clinically and in research, further abstracts the human condition to the cellular, biochemical, or structural level (Feinstein, 1973) and excludes the psychological, social, and cultural dimensions of life. However, quantitative research is obviously applicable in studies of physiology, pathology, biochemistry, pharmacology, microbiology, and other basic sciences, and in large-scale epidemiological surveys. By contrast with ethnography, positivism "moves from idea to data instead of from data to idea"(Peacock, 1986).

However, from an anthropological perspective, scientific empiricism can be regarded also as culture-bound; that is, it is shaped by, and expresses, certain cultural and social assumptions of Western society. As Peacock (1986) remarks, "a fact is a percept viewed through a frame of reference." This frame of reference, which produces the fact or datum, is in turn the product of a particular cultural time and place. In Eisenberg's (1977) view, "models are ways of constructing reality, ways of imposing meaning on the chaos of the phenomenal world. . . . Once in place, models act to generate their own verification by excluding phenomena outside the frame of reference the user employs." Models are thus indispensable, but "hazardous because they can be mistaken for reality itself rather than as but one way of organizing that reality." Furthermore, Western numbering systems and statistics are culture-bound, since other cultures employ different systems of numbering (e.g., without the emphasis on 100 as a crucial unit of analysis, as in percentage calculations). Graphs, diagrams, and mathematical models can be regarded as culturally determined ideograms or symbolic representations of the phenomenological world; they employ concepts of space, time, and significance that arise from modern industrial culture (Littlewood, 1984). The use of questionnaires, as in sociological surveys, is also a culture-bound research instrument: The framing of experience into specific questions, the imposed order of questions, and the linear structure of narrative they imply, may all be inappropriate for certain social or cultural groups. Other forms of questionnaires, including multiple-choice questions and questions with only a limited number of possible answers (e.g., "is the pain—better/the same/worse?") also impose a culturally specific and limited mode of enquiry on the objects of the study. Finally, the mere presence of the researcher may alter the phenomena under study, a fact increasingly recognized in modern science (Snow, 1981).

The ethnographic, qualitative approach, by contrast, is appropriate for research into the following:

- lay health beliefs, perceptions of illness, and the patient's explanatory models that underlie these (Kleinman, 1980);
- the meanings that patients give to particular symptoms, diagnostic labels, tests and treatments (Kleinman, 1983);
- patients' religions, world-views and cultural explanations of misfortune, including ill health (Helman, 1984a);

- health-related beliefs and behaviors (including family health culture), as well as health needs in the community, as part of research underlying community-oriented primary care (Madison, 1983);
- the relationship between culturally determined behavior and the incidence of certain organic diseases, as in the case of kuru (Gadjusek, 1973);
- doctor-patient consultations and communication (Helman, 1981);
- studies of the social, cultural, and economic contexts of ill health, medical diagnosis, and medical treatment (including power relations, gender issues, economic factors, and design of facilities);
- institutional organization and subcultures of medical institutions, such as clinics, nursing homes, and hospitals (Goffman, 1961); and
- comparisons of different national systems of health care, and allocation of resources in relation to their core cultural values (Payer, 1988).

The usefulness of the ethnographic approach is limited by a number of factors:

- it is labor-intensive, and more time is needed to conduct interviews (which may have to be recorded, transcribed, and analyzed) and collect other ethnographic data;
- it requires researchers specially trained in ethnographic techniques;
- it is suitable mainly for studies on smaller groups of subjects;
- it does not use the random sampling method as does qualitative research, and thus informants may not be typical of the group and may provide different information;
- there is the possibility of observer error and disagreement among observers, the "Rashomon Effect" (Heider, 1988), since the presence of the observer may influence the study; and
- it is unsuitable for large-scale surveys and research into physiological phenomena.

The Scope of Qualitative Research in Primary Care

In the section above I have mentioned a number of applications of qualitative research methods, many of which are relevant to primary care. It should be noted that a good physician will already be a good ethnographer, since there are similarities between the techniques employed in both spheres. These techniques include:

- the use of the case-history method in illustrating general phenomena by reference to a particular case;
- the taking of personal and social medical histories;
- psychotherapeutic techniques, which allow patients to express their beliefs, fears, and hopes;
- the participant observation that any physician in a community carries out, gradually building up a picture of the life of a particular patient, family, or community;
- the exploration of beliefs and behaviors in daily life and whether they are protective of health or pathogenic (e.g., smoking, drinking, drug abuse, promiscuity);
- identifying discrepancies between observed, measurable data about patients and their stated version of their own behavior (e.g., abnormal liver function tests or raised blood-alcohol level in a patient who denies alcohol intake);
- observing the natural history of ill health and illness careers over time; and
- treating the patient within the context of his or her own family, and treating the family itself as a collective patient or "system" (Christie-Seely, 1981).

In addition to studies of illness, explanatory models, health beliefs and behaviors, doctor-patient communication, social networks, and the role played in these by social, cultural, religious, and ethnic factors, qualitative research is also relevant to the study of what I term "family health culture." This conceives of the family as a small-scale society (though family structures differ cross-culturally; Fox, 1967), with its own "subculture" of beliefs and behaviors, which may be either protective of health or pathogenic. These may include specific dietary patterns; dress; gender roles; child-rearing practices; family myths and rituals; attitudes towards alcohol, tobacco or drugs; patterns of symptomatology; health-seeking behavior; attitudes toward ill health and other misfortunes; attitudes toward physicians and their treatments; self-medication; leisure pursuits and hobbies; attitudes toward sexuality, menstruation, and pregnancy; personal hygiene; resolution of conflicts; and life-cycle changes and rituals. Family health culture can best be examined by a long-term ethnographic approach carried out by the physician or by a trained assistant.

Qualitative Research Projects in Primary Care

Research projects in primary care should usually employ a combination of quantitative and qualitative methodologies (Crane & Angrosino, 1974; Like, Rogers, & McGoldrick, 1988; Mull, 1985). However, both types of techniques should be accompanied by an ethnographically informed awareness of their limitations.

Research can be carried out by a physician, nurse, paramedic, social scientist, or member of the local community trained for this task. To some extent, the choice of researcher may influence the data that can be obtained. Research venues can include the doctor's office, a hospital ward or clinic, the patient's home, or other settings in the community. Each requires a different approach, since each "context" influences the types of communication possible in that setting (Hall, 1983; Helman, 1984b) and what is said, heard, or ignored by each party.

There are a number of basic methods in qualitative research that are relevant to primary health care. These are:

1. *Questionnaires:* These can be structured or semistructured, which may be directed at a specific question (e.g., dietary habits and taboos during pregnancy) or at a wider problem (e.g., beliefs about the origin, significance, and treatment of heart disease). Even if structured, the questionnaire should include at least one open-ended question (e.g., "Why did you get ill?"), which may reveal more complex, "high-context" explanations not revealed by the other questions. Questions may be asked in a particular order, but the interviewees may not reply in that same order. Answers may have to be transcribed into the questionnaires after the interview has ended.

2. *Ethnography:* This entails fieldwork by a participant observer, with the researcher being a "fly on the wall," blending in as much as possible with the environment. Physicians may be well placed to be such invisible observers in a variety of medical situations, especially among their own colleagues. Data are collected by observation and recorded in written notes, tape, or video recordings.

3. *Interviews:* These are open-ended, and conducted with "native informants" who are members of the community or family. They are usually tape-recorded and help form hypotheses for further investigation.

4. *Family interviews:* Based on techniques of family therapy (Di-Nicola, 1986; Minuchin, Rosman, & Baker, 1978), these examine family health culture and may involve the use of genograms (Like, Rogers, & McGoldrick, 1988, pp. 407-412) or compilation of a "family health tree" (Prince-Embury, 1984).

5. *Video and audio tape-recordings, photographs:* These facilitate studies of specific events (e.g., doctor-patient consultations, medical rituals, behavior in clinic waiting rooms, body language of patients or health professionals).

6. *Narratives:* These are autobiographical accounts of ill health, surgical operations, diagnostic procedures, or doctor-patient interactions. They are usually recorded or written down by the interviewee.

7. *Data collection:* Usually consisting of physiological information (e.g., blood pressure levels, urinary catecholamines, height and weight, caloric intake, hemoglobin level), this may include written information such as previous research literature, census reports, or data on disease incidence.

8. *Genealogies:* Collected from informants and cross-checked if possible with written sources, these are useful in gaining an understanding of kinship patterns, inheritance of symptoms and family health culture, and hereditary diseases.

9. *Projective techniques:* These are similar to the use of the Rorschach and other tests in psychology. Subjects are shown films or photographs (e.g., of an individual showing typical signs of a disease), or are given written or spoken vignettes of a certain cluster of symptoms, and are asked to interpret these in terms of their personal and cultural perspectives on ill health.

10. *Examination of written or printed material:* These include studies of printed text, newspaper articles, books, family diaries, letters, and records, as well as family photographs.

Examples of clinically relevant research projects that can be carried out in a primary care setting are outlined below.

1. *Collection of explanatory models:* Studies of lay beliefs about the origin, significance, prognosis, and appropriate treatment of ill health or other misfortunes (Calnan, 1987; Cassell, 1978; Helman,

1981; Kleinman et al., 1978). Such data are usually "snapshots" of beliefs at a particular time and place, and follow-up studies may have to be carried out. This is an important technique in understanding illness, noncompliance, and self-treatment. Explanatory models for the same condition can be compared among different social or ethnic groups. Examples include Blumhagen (1980) on hypertension and Helman (1978) on colds, chills, and fever.

2. *Comparisons of disease and illness perspectives:* Studies of medical and lay explanatory models, and how they agree or differ. These are also "snapshot" studies, but they are useful for identifying and quantifying communication problems between doctor and patient (Helman, 1985a). They should be related to the time and context in which the communication takes place. Examples include studies done on differing perspectives on psychosomatic disorders (Helman, 1985a), child-bearing (Graham & Oakley, 1986), surgical treatment (Cay, Philip, Small, Neilson, & Henderson, 1975) and *nervios* in Costa Rica (Low, 1988).

3. *Semantic network studies:* Based on the work of Good and Good (1981) and Good (1977), these are similar to psychoanalytic free-association techniques and usually require several interviews. They examine the web of meanings associated with a particular symptom, body part, diagnostic label, folk illness category, or type of treatment. Each of these may carry a range of symbolic meanings for the patient (moral, social, or psychological), linking the suffering experienced to a wider context. Examples include Good (1977) on Iranian heart distress and Blumhagen (1980) on hypertension.

4. *Doctor-patient consultations:* These are analyzed after being recorded on video or audiotape. This is a "low context" technique, but can be combined with techniques 1-3 above for a fuller picture. It can also be used to analyze nonverbal behavior between doctor and patient, and the "messages" conveyed by the physical setting in which the consultation takes place. Examples include Byrne and Long (1976) on medical consultations, and Pietroni (1976) on nonverbal behavior in the doctor's office.

5. *Impact studies:* Studies of the psychological, behavioral, physiological, economic, and social impacts on individuals and their families or communities, of a particular consultation, diagnostic label, diagnostic test, or medical treatment. May include use of the Sickness Impact Profile questionnaire (Bergner & Gilson, 1980).

6. *Studies of body imagery:* Studies of patients' knowledge of the structure and function of the body, their indigenous models of physiology, and how these relate to their interpretations of symptoms. Examples are beliefs about the location of organs (Boyle, 1970), bodily perceptions after surgery (Tait & Ascher, 1955), and Ayurvedic models of physiology (Obeyesekere, 1977).

7. *Ethnography of a clinical event:* Studies of a particular clinical event such as a consultation, diagnostic procedure, or surgical operation, where *all* participants in the event (e.g., doctor, patient, nurse, receptionist, technician, spouse, relative) are interviewed, and their accounts, plus the observer's, are analyzed and compared so that the totality of the event, the differing perspectives on it, and why these occurred can be understood. An example of this is a study (Helman, 1985b) of the impact on a patient with "pseudo-angina" of the differing perspectives of five physicians who treated him.

8. *Narratives of health and illness:* Collections of autobiographical accounts of ill health or other clinical events are written down or taped, so that an understanding of how such "stories of sickness" (Brody, 1987) shape and give meaning to the human experience of suffering may be gained.

9. *Studies of medical pluralism:* Studies of nonmedical forms of health care and advice in the "hidden health care system," before or after consultation with a physician. Examples include McGuire (1988) on ritual healing in the suburban United States, Scott (1974) on different healing systems in Miami, Levy (1982) on self-help groups in Britain, and Elliott-Binns (1973) on self-treatment in England.

10. *Collection of oral medical folklore:* Studies of inherited, traditional forms of self-treatment, such as "old wives' tales" (Chamberlain, 1981). Examples include Snow (1977) on American menstrual folklore.

11. *Ethnography of a medical institution:* Participant-observation studies of a hospital, clinic, ward, doctor's office, or diagnostic procedure. Examples include Goffman (1961) on asylums, Katz (1981) on surgical rituals, Hahn (1985) on internist behavior, and Lella and Pawluch (1988) on medical students' experiences of dissection.

12. *Ethnography of a folk healer:* Participation-observation studies of the clinical approach of traditional, folk, or alternative healers to their patients, with the aim of understanding how these differ

from biomedicine, and the strengths or weaknesses of this approach. Examples include Kleinman (1983) on Taiwanese healers, Finkler (1985) on Mexican spiritualist healers, and Mull (1988) on a traditional Islamic healer.

13. *Studies of family health culture:* Long-term ethnographic studies of particular families, which may include the use of genograms (Like et al., 1888), family health trees (Prince-Embury, 1984), and some of the concepts and techniques of family therapy (DiNicola, 1986; Minuchin et al., 1978). Examples include Minuchin et al. (1978) on "psychosomatic families" and McGoldrick, Pearce, and Giordano (1982) on ethnicity in family therapy. Such studies may need to include physiological and epidemiological data.

14. *Ethnography of patient populations:* Studies of small circumscribed groups with their own subculture, such as Burr on urban drug addicts (Burr, 1984).

15. *Studies of social networks:* Ethnographic studies of an individual's or family's significant social networks, and how these relate to health, disease, illness, and self-treatment. Examples include Elliott-Binns (1973) on nonmedical health advice, and McKinlay (1980) on networks and help-seeking behavior.

Conclusion

In this chapter I have outlined the contributions of qualitative techniques to research in primary health care. I have also discussed some of the concepts from medical anthropology that underlie this approach. Qualitative research is particularly useful in studying why people act in particular ways and in investigating the relationship of beliefs and behavior to one another. It is the research technique of choice in studying how ethnic, religious, or social variables influence health, disease, illness, and help-seeking behavior. More positivist, quantitative research methodologies are also useful, but often exclude these dimensions and are themselves influenced by the cultural context in which they are used. Qualitative research is also subject to certain limitations and is not appropriate for all situations in primary care, but it can usefully be combined with quantitative research to attain a fuller picture.

Primary care and family physicians have unique opportunities and many of the skills necessary to carry out such research. The aim of the research should be to facilitate primary health care that is humane, efficient, culturally appropriate, cost-effective, and suited to the needs of both patient and physician.

References

Bergner, M., & Gilson, B. S. (1980). The sickness impact profile: The relevance of social science to medicine. In L. Eisenberg & A. Kleinman (Eds.), *The relevance of social science for medicine* (pp. 135-150). Dordrecht: Reidel.

Blumhagen, D. (1980). Hypertension: A folk illness with a medical name.*Culture, Medicine and Psychiatry, 4,* 197-227.

Boyle, C. M. (1970). Difference between patients' and doctors' interpretation of some common medical terms. *British Medical Journal, 2,* 286-289.

Brody, H. (1987). *Stories of sickness.* New Haven: Yale University Press.

Burr, A. (1984). The ideologies of despair: A symbolic interpretation of punks' and skinheads' usage of barbiturates. *Social Sciences in Medicine, 9,* 929-938.

Byrne, P. S., & Long, B. E. L. (1976). *Doctors talking to patients.* London: HMSO.

Calnan, M. (1987). *Health and illness: The lay perspective.* London: Tavistock.

Cassell, E. J. (1978). *The healer's art: A new approach to the doctor-patient relationship.* Harmondsworth: Penguin.

Cay, E. L., Philip, A. E., Small, W. P., Neilson, J., & Henderson, M. A. (1975). Patients' assessment of the result of surgery for peptic ulcer. *Lancet, 1,* 29-31.

Chamberlain, M. (1981). *Old wives' tales.* London: Virago.

Christie-Seely, J. (1981). Teaching the family system concept in family medicine. *Journal of Family Practice, 13,* 391-401.

Crane, J. S., & Angrosino, M. V. (1974). *Field projects in anthropology: A student handbook.* Glenview, IL: Scott, Foresman.

DiNicola, V. F. (1986). Beyond Babel: Family therapy as cultural translation. *International Journal of Family Therapy, 7,* 179-191.

Eisenberg, L. (1977). Disease and illness: Distinctions between professional and popular ideas of sickness. *Culture, Medicine and Psychiatry, 1,* 9-23.

Elliott-Binns, C. P. (1973). An analysis of lay medicine. *Journal of the Royal College of General Practice, 23,* 255-264.

Feinstein, A. R. (1973). An analysis of diagnostic reasoning; Part I and II. *Yale Journal of Biology and Medicine, 15,* 583-616.

Finkler, K. (1985). *Spiritualist healers in Mexico.* South Hadley: Bergin & Garvey.

Foster, G. M., & Anderson, B. G. (1978). *Medical anthropology.* New York: John Wiley.

Fox, R. (1967). *Kinship and marriage.* Harmondsworth: Penguin.

Gadjusek, D. C. (1973). Kuru in the New Guinea Highlands. In J. D. Spillane (Ed.), *Tropical neurology* (pp. 377-383). New York: Oxford University Press.

Goffman, E. (1961). *Asylums.* Harmondsworth: Penguin.

Good, B. (1977). The heart of what's the matter: The semantics of illness in Iran. *Culture, Medicine and Psychiatry, 1,* 25-58.

Good, B. J., & Good M. J. D. (1981). The meaning of symptoms: A cultural hermeneutic model for clinical practice. In L. Eisenberg & A. Kleinman (Eds.), *The relevance of social science for medicine* (pp. 165-196). Dordrecht: Reidel.

Graham, H., & Oakley, A. (1986). Competing ideologies of reproduction: Medical and maternal perspectives on pregnancy. In C. Currer & M. Stacey (Eds.), *Concepts of health, illness and disease* (pp. 99-135). Leamington Spa: Berg.

Hahn, R. A. (1985). A world of internal medicine: Portrait of an internist. In R. A. Hahn & A. D. Gaines (Eds.), *Physicians of Western medicine* (pp. 51-111). Dordrecht: Reidel.

Hall, E. T. (1969). *The hidden dimension.* New York: Anchor.

Hall, E. T. (1977). *Beyond culture.* New York: Anchor.

Hall, E. T. (1983). *The dance of life.* New York: Anchor.

Harwood, A. (Ed.). (1981). *Ethnicity and medical care.* Cambridge, MA: Harvard University Press.

Heider, K. G. (1988). The Rashomon effect: Ethnographers disagree. *American Anthropology, 90,* 73-81.

Helman, C. G. (1978). "Feed a cold, starve a fever": Folk models of infection in an English suburban community, and their relation to medical treatment. *Culture, Medicine and Psychiatry, 2,* 107-137.

Helman, C. G. (1981). Disease versus illness in general practice. *Journal of the Royal College of General Practice, 31,* 548-552.

Helman, C. G. (1984a). *Culture, health and illness: An introduction for health professionals.* Bristol: Wright.

Helman, C. G. (1984b). The role of context in primary care. *Journal of the Royal College of General Practice, 34,* 547-550.

Helman, C. G. (1985a). Communication in primary care: The role of patient and practitioner explanatory models. *Social Sciences in Medicine, 20,* 923-931.

Helman, C. G. (1985b). Disease and pseudo-disease: A case history of pseudo-angina. In R. A. Hahn & A. D. Gaines (Eds.), *Physicians of Western medicine* (pp. 269-292). Dordrecht: Reidel.

Helman, C. G. (1987). General practice and the hidden health care system. *Journal of the Royal Society of Medicine, 80,* 738-740.

Helman, C. G. (1990). Cultural factors in health and illness. In B. R. McAvoy & L. Donaldson (Eds.), *Health care for Asians* (pp. 17-27). Oxford, UK: Oxford University Press.

Kaplan, A. (1968). Positivism. In D. L. Sill (Ed.), *International encyclopaedia of the social sciences* (Vol. 12) (pp. 389-395). New York: Macmillan Free Press.

Katz, P. (1981). Ritual in the operating room. *Ethnology, 20,* 335-350.

Keesing, R. M. (1981). *Cultural anthropology: A contemporary perspective.* New York: Holt, Rinehart & Winston.

Kleinman, A. (1980). *Patient and healers in the context of culture.* Berkeley: University of California Press.

Kleinman, A. (1983). The cultural meanings and social uses of illness. *Journal of Family Practice, 16,* 539-545.

Kleinman, A., Eisenberg, L., & Good, B. (1978). Culture, illness and care: Clinical lessons from anthropologic and cross-cultural research. *Annals of Internal Medicine, 88,* 251-258.

Landy, D. (Ed.). (1977). *Culture, disease and healing.* New York: Macmillan.

Lella, J. W., & Pawluch, D. (1988). Medical students and the cadaver in social and cultural context. In M. Lock & D. R. Gordon (Eds.), *Biomedicine examined* (pp. 125-153). Dordrecht: Kluwer.

Levy, L. (1982). Mutual support groups in Great Britain. *Social Sciences in Medicine, 16*, 1265-1275.

Like, R. C., Rogers, J., & McGoldrick, M. (1988). Reading and interpreting genograms: A systematic approach. *Journal of Family Practice, 26*, 407-412.

Like, R. C., & Steiner, R. P. (1986). Medical anthropology and the family physician. *Family Medicine, 18*, 87-92.

Littlewood, R. (1984). The individual articulation of shared symbols. *Journal of Operational Psychology, 15*, 17-24.

Low, S. M. (1988). Medical practice in response to a folk illness: The diagnosis and treatment of *nervios* in Costa Rica. In M. Lock & D. R. Gordon (Eds.), *Biomedicine examined* (pp. 415-438). Dordrecht: Kluwer.

McGoldrick, M., Pearce, J. K., & Giordano, J. (Eds.). (1982). *Ethnicity and family therapy*. New York: Guilford Press.

McGuire, M. B. (1988). *Ritual healing in suburban America*. New Brunswick, NJ: Rutgers University Press.

McKinlay, J. B. (1980). Social network influences on morbid episodes and the career of help-seeking. In L. Eisenberg & A. Kleinman (Eds.), *The relevance of social science for medicine* (pp. 77-107). Dordrecht: Reidel.

Madison, D. L. (1983). The case for community-oriented primary care. *Journal of the American Medical Association, 249*, 1279-1282.

Mares, P., Henley, A., & Baxter, C. (1985). *Health care in multiracial Britain*. Cambridge, UK: Health Education Council.

Minuchin, S., Rosman, B. L., & Baker, L. (1978). *Psychosomatic families*. Cambridge, MA: Harvard University Press.

More anthropology and less sleep for medical students.(1980). *British Medical Journal, 281*, 1662.

Mull, J. D. (1985). Medical anthropology: The art and science of people studying people. *Family Practice Research, 5*, 67-78.

Mull J. D. (1988). Light in the afternoon. *Journal of the American Medical Association, 260*, 393.

Obeyesekere, G. (1977). The theory and practice of Ayurvedic medicine. *Culture, Medicine and Psychiatry, 1*, 155-181.

Payer, L. (1988). *Medicine and culture*. New York: Henry Holt.

Peacock, J. L. (1986). *The anthropological lens: Harsh light, soft focus*. Cambridge, UK: Cambridge University Press.

Pietroni, P. (1976). Non-verbal communication in the general-practice surgery. In B. Tanner (Ed.), *Language and communication in general practice* (pp. 162-179). London: Hodder & Stoughton.

Prince-Embury, S. (1984). The family health tree: A form for identifying physical symptom patterns within the family. *Journal of Family Practice, 18*, 75-81.

Scott, C. S. (1974). Health and healing practices among five ethnic groups in Miami. *Public Health Reports, 89*, 524-532.

Snow, C. P. (1981). *The physicists*. London: Macmillan.

Snow, L. S. (1977). Modern day menstrual folklore. *Journal of the American Medical Association, 237*, 2736-2739.

Tait, C. D., & Ascher, R. C. (1955). Inside-of-the-body test. *Psychosomatic Medicine, 17,* 139-148.

Tolstoy, L. (1930). *What is art* (A. Maude, Trans.). London: Oxford University Press.

Warwick, I., Aggleton, P., & Homand, H. (1988). Young people's health beliefs and AIDS. In P. Aggleton & H. Homans (Eds.), *Social aspects of AIDS* (pp. 106-125). London: Falmer.

9 Qualitative Research in Primary Care

HOWARD BRODY

Introduction

In clinical medicine, qualitative research includes case reports, nonstatistical analyses of one's clinical practice or experience, and reports of structured patient interviews. Other disciplines that may study problems arising from clinical medicine, and which are normally seen as engaging primarily in qualitative research, include some social sciences (such as anthropology and certain methodological approaches within psychology and sociology), philosophy and ethics, history, literary criticism, linguistics, religious studies, and law. This list is, of course, hardly exhaustive.

Ideally, a chapter on this topic would offer an extensive literature review of each of the above disciplines as applied to primary care medicine, and would suggest standards for evaluating the quality of research carried out in each. However, it should be obvious that such a task is well beyond the capacity of most scholars, to say nothing of the poor physician. I will therefore address myself to a much more modest effort. First, I will offer a framework for viewing the importance of qualitative methods generally in clinical medicine and understanding what they can add to a body of research that is pursued only in quantitative terms. Next, I will try to illustrate this framework and the complementary nature of qualitative and quantitative methods that it suggests by describing in some detail a research project that I have recently been planning along with some colleagues at

Michigan State University. While this project has yet to be carried out, I believe that it has some illustrative features that make it a good exploratory example.

Ways of Knowing in Medicine

In our age any discussion of qualitative methods in medical research must begin with a defense of using them at all. Not only is medical research widely viewed as being synonymous with quantitative approaches; but also many would charge that the reason that research in primary care has low status and priority within the biomedical establishment is its past reliance almost exclusively on qualitative methods, and that only a strong and sustained quantitative turn can reverse its fortunes.

To respond to this implied skepticism, I wish to counter with a strong devil's advocate position. I would argue that not only can qualitative methods supplement and expand the research insights of the better accepted quantitative techniques, but also that the over-reliance on the latter, and the fact that they are seen as somehow having a privileged status because of the certainty of the knowledge they generate, is based on a myth. Western thinkers fell in love with that myth in the seventeenth century, for reasons that seemed good then but are hardly applicable to choices we must make today. Philosophers, increasingly, and scientists and physicians, gradually, are beginning to see that myth for what it really is.

The myth of quantitative supremacy is actually a more recent chapter in a very old philosophical debate in Western culture between advocates of fundamentally different approaches to human knowledge. A nice description of this debate is given in a recent insightful work by Jonsen and Toulmin on the history of moral discourse (Jonsen & Toulmin, 1988). While the authors focus on ethics, the same features they point out are true also of science, and indeed they use clinical medicine frequently as an example of the sort of practical problem-solving activity to which applied ethics may fruitfully be compared.

The debate can be seen as having started between Plato and Aristotle. Plato thought fundamentally that to have knowledge worthy of the name meant having special insights into truths or concepts that had two important features: first, they held true universally and eternally; and second, the conclusions drawn from them had the force of logical necessity. Aristotle had a basically different view of human knowledge. He agreed that some spheres of knowledge allowed for the clarity and purity associated with Plato's eternal forms, which were, in an important way, aspects or extensions of geometry. But he also insisted that other aspects of human activity allowed only for knowledge that was probabilistic and context-specific. Besides truths that held universally and of necessity, he allowed for those that held in certain cases insofar as certain conditions were met, but which might not hold if any of a number of exceptional conditions were encountered. Aristotle argued that knowledge of this latter type was still knowledge, and that it would bear a considerable degree of rational analysis and method. He refused to categorize knowledge as first-class and second-class; instead he categorized different sorts of human activity and inquiry according to the degree of certainty or probability, universality, and concreteness that each would allow. While ethics is clearly an example of the concrete, probabilistic sort of knowledge, Aristotle also thought that the biological, and what we would call today the social sciences, fell into that category, along with rhetoric and politics.

Aristotle had the most influence upon the science and ethics of the medieval period, but this was challenged in the seventeenth century. A pivotal figure may have been the French scientist and mathematician Blaise Pascal, who was responsible not only for several advances in mathematical methods but also for a scathing attack upon casuistry, the dominant mode of practical ethical analysis used by the Catholic church up to that time. Both medieval science (what there was of it) and medieval ethics had slipped into many sloppy habits and indeed had a lot to answer for. But Pascal saw himself, in his attacks, going well beyond simply purging an Aristotelian approach of its weaknesses and misuses and re-establishing it on a stronger footing. Instead, he was effectively rejecting Aristotelianism for Platonism. Tired of the murkiness of medieval scholasticism, and enthralled by developments in mathematics brought about by his contemporaries such as Descartes, Pascal felt that the only salvation for human reason lay in the search for eternal, universal laws of both science and ethics. Like Plato, he convinced himself that because geometry was so elegant and pure, it simply had to be the case that all human activities were enough like geometry that geometry-like axioms, theorems, and laws could be formulated to explain them.

Basically, Western intellectual thought has pursued Platonism ever since, even though physics, usually thought to be the most mathematical of the natural sciences, has taken a decidedly non-Platonic turn since 1905. Of late, growing philosophical critique has been aimed at the basic myth that underlies this choice of worldviews—that just because we happen to be enchanted with geometry, the world has to be enough like geometry in all of its aspects so that geometrical methods can always be used to explain everything that is of interest to us. All through the period in which this myth has held sway, there seem to have been sufficient successes of the geometric method to ensure that it would be viewed as superior. It is only in historical hindsight, with the aid of philosophical scrutiny, that the amazing successes of this method can be shown to have relied on sweeping and arbitrary assumptions about which phenomena are pertinent and interesting and which are not. It is fairly easy to "prove" that quantitative methods are a superior way of gaining knowledge about the world, as long as we agree beforehand by social convention that we will regard as questions worth asking only those that can easily be answered by such methods.

An alternative approach to human knowledge, which breaks free of the Platonic geometry myth, has been provided by the psychologist Jerome Bruner (1986). Bruner reviews a good deal of recent psychological data to argue that the most basic way human beings have of making sense of their experience in the world is the narrative mode. Put simply, we make sense of events by telling stories about them and we depict and construct our relations with things and with other people by placing them in various ways within the stories of our lives and our culture. To tell these stories is to frame theories about temporal relationships, causation, and human agency; to criticize stories and to offer alternative ones is to evaluate which of the competing theories best accord with the available empirical data.

Bruner goes on to point out that as we get away from the very basic mode of story-telling or narrative, we encounter other, more formal and sophisticated ways of framing and testing theories about the world, including quantitative scientific methods. But he insists that these are ultimately derived from the more basic, narrative mode. For all its power and precision, quantitative science or mathematics is simply another way of telling stories about our place in the world: what came first, what came next, and why things happened the way they did.

I believe that this reminder of the fundamental role of the narrative mode is important to us for several reasons. First, we must note that one of the things that many (but not all) of the so-called qualitative methods from the social sciences and the humanities have in common is the employment of a specifically narrative approach to explaining events. In particular, these methods take seriously the way that subjects of observation themselves try to make sense of events, the stories they tell about them, and the meanings that they attribute to them. When we use quantitative methods, we decide what we are going to count and what we are going to leave out, and the subjects' frameworks of thoughts or meaning are irrelevant to the experiment. In contrast, if we use, say, an ethnographic method, we have no choice but to ask the subjects what meaning *they* attribute to the events and to listen to their stories before we try to attach meanings of our own. As Kuzel (1986) has noted in a useful review of the methods of naturalistic inquiry, any sort of social science, including the quantitative variety, might be a *study of people*; but an ethnographic or naturalistic approach is rather a means of *learning from people*. In the former case, we construct narratives about people to explain what they do, and those narratives might or might not be recognizable or make sense to the subjects themselves. When we employ a qualitative approach and learn from people, we must first and foremost attend to the stories that are their primary way of making sense of their own experiences for themselves.

In the context of this book, it should be remembered that a healthy utilization of the narrative approach is one of the features that distinguishes primary care medicine from subspecialty practice (Herbert, 1988). In a powerful critique of the dominant biomedical model, George Engel (1988) has argued that the most basic mark of good science is careful and accurate data gathering, and the patient's own story of an illness is the necessary starting point for any scientific medical inquiry. If the primary care physician takes care to set the patient at ease, asks appropriately supportive and open-ended questions, and generally uses the physician-patient relationship as a tool toward better and more complete narration, then he or she is being *more scientific* than the subspecialist, who is often tempted to short-circuit the history and reach immediately for the endoscope or the imaging device. In other words, a healthy respect for the value of narrative as a mode of careful, thoughtful inquiry ought to be an attribute that primary care medicine shares with the qualitative humanities and social sciences (Brody, 1987).

To summarize what has necessarily been an extremely sketchy account thus far, I contend that Aristotle had a better grasp than did Plato of the complexities of the world we seek to explain and of the many different sorts of questions we wish to ask about it, each requiring in turn different methods of investigation. Almost always, when someone proposes that only one method or set of methods ought to explain everything about the world, we discover upon further reflection that this individual is really saying that only a very narrow set of questions is worth asking. Many sciences can proceed, and indeed can make great strides, by severely limiting the questions to be asked and then attacking those questions with depth and precision. However, it is much less likely that a field such as primary care medicine will yield to this sort of narrow approach, because the questions that need to be asked often emerge with the ongoing practice and cannot be specified or limited in advance.

This suggests in turn that both quantitative and qualitative methods have appropriate applications in primary care research, even though in theory the latter better reflects the unique defining features of primary care.

A Research Case Study

As I can offer no rules for when qualitative methods will be most fruitful in primary care research or how they can best be combined and coordinated with quantitative methods, I will turn instead to a fairly detailed description of an ongoing research effort, the most important component of which has yet to be carried out. If I am successful in describing the rationale for the research design, it may serve as a helpful illustration.

True to my advocacy of a narrative method, I begin by telling the story of the origins of this research effort. I became interested in the placebo effect as a subject for a doctoral dissertation in philosophy, in hopes of using it to illuminate the medical implications of the mind-body relationship (Brody, 1980). This led me to read a good deal of literature on the placebo effect, most of which was of the quantitative variety. I approached this literature from the standpoint of one sort of qualitative research—analytic philosophy. I sought to define unclear terms, offer useful distinctions, and generally to construct logical arguments that would lead to interesting conclusions.

This qualitative, analytic assessment of the literature led me to two conclusions. First, I felt convinced that the placebo effect was a very broad phenomenon that was in important ways dependent upon the entire context of the physician-patient relationship, including the cultural belief systems within which that encounter occurred, as well as the personal belief systems of the two individuals involved. Second, I felt convinced that the explanatory theories that had appeared so far, such as classical conditioning, transference, expectation, and suggestibility, were much narrower in focus than the phenomenon they sought to explain. It occurred to me that I might propose an empirically testable theory that was more comprehensive than its predecessors.

My theoretical model turned out to be heavily dependent upon two qualitative studies of the physician-patient relationship: an anthropological paper by Adler and Hammett (1973), and a reflective book on clinical practice by Cassell (1976). I dubbed it the "meaning model" because it postulated that a positive (or negative) placebo effect would occur when the meaning of the illness experience was changed for the patient in a positive (or negative) manner. In turn, this meaning was postulated to hinge on three major elements, essentially interconnected but theoretically distinguishable: first, whether an explanation was offered that made sense in terms of the patient's accepted worldview; second, whether the patient experienced the immediate social group as expressing care and concern; and third, whether the patient achieved a sense of mastery or control over the symptoms or the illness.

This model or theory appeared to me to be empirically testable, and I recalled little in the medical literature on placebos that directly contradicted it. Moreover, one particular study seemed to validate it: This study showed the effect of an anesthesiologist's supportive and informative preoperative visit on the extent of postoperative pain and need for medication. That is, the authors of this study seem to have implicitly hit upon a similar theory, which their data tended to confirm (Egbert, Battit, Welch, & Bartlett, 1964). In conclusion, I had derived a theory that could be tested, both by qualitative and (I thought) quantitative methods, from a qualitative analysis of largely quantitatively derived data. (It might be worth noting here that a peculiarity of the medical literature on placebo phenomena is that a great deal of what is known about them comes not from studies of the placebo effect but from something else; when placebos are used as controls in research, interesting findings in the control group may be a totally unintended consequence of the original research.)

Over the next several years I happily observed the publication of studies that appeared to offer further confirmation of the meaning model and which, unlike the older anesthesia study, began to break down the positive response into separate elements and to study them as discrete contributors. These studies were all quantitative in design (Bass, Buck, Turner, Dickie, Pratt, & Robinson, 1983; Greenfield, Kaplan, & Ware, 1985; The Headache Study Group, 1986). My own work, however, continued along the same qualitative track and took the form of further philosophical analyses of the physician-patient relationship and the importance of its symbolic dimensions (Brody, 1987). This additional qualitative work served to convince me further that the meaning model was sound. Unfortunately, I felt more and more like a spectator as I waited for others to chance upon a model like mine and subject it to experimental scrutiny. It seemed to me that, as a primary care academic physician, I had some duty to put my money where my mouth was and try to design a study that was intended explicitly to test the meaning model.

I had a good many thoughts about this, but what finally brought them into focus was the chance discovery that a teaching colleague of mine, a psychophysiologist, had been doing work with an ambulatory blood-pressure monitoring device, for which he had designed a simplified but informative computerized log. By his method, one could plot a subject's blood pressure at 15-minute intervals over 24 hours and determine at each of those reading times the activity level, mood, and substance ingestion of the subject (VanEgeren & Madarasmi, 1988). His interest in using this device to study the placebo effect in a group of mild hypertensives led to a study design that seemed especially promising for teasing out one particular element of the meaning model.

We proposed to enroll a group of mild or borderline hypertensives and randomize them, according to a two-by-two cell design, into four groups. One study variable would be the extent to which response to medication (or placebo) was influenced by how well the explanation for medication efficacy matched the subject's preexisting preferred model for hypertension and its treatment. For this aspect of the study, we would employ qualitative, anthropological, or ethnographic methods to interview a representative group of hypertensive patients drawn from the same population. We would hope to find, as Helman (1981) did in studying patient views of benzodiazepine efficacy, three to five discrete and recurring models or concepts of how antihypertensives work. From this qualitative preliminary study would come two outputs essential for further research: first, a brief questionnaire or structured interview protocol that would allow us to classify future subjects according to their preferred model; and second, videotapes in which a physician would explain the efficacy of the antihypertensive to be employed in this study, in the terms and concepts peculiar to each of the explanatory models.

The second study variable, according to which subjects would also be randomized, would be the administration of either an angiotensin converting-enzyme inhibitor or a placebo (in double-blind fashion).

We proposed that the study would proceed in the following sequence. After being found medically suitable and after giving informed consent (which would be quite detailed regarding the drug-versus-placebo design and the nature of the ambulatory device, but deliberately vague regarding the explanatory model component), subjects would receive the questionnaire or undergo a brief interview, and would be classified according to their preferred explanatory model. Next, the first baseline 24-hour blood-pressure recording would be made. The subjects would then, in single-blind fashion, be randomized to view either the "matching" or a randomly chosen "mismatched" videotape that explained the workings of the ACE inhibitor in language either fully consistent with, or else at odds with, the patient's own preferred explanatory model. They would next receive (in double-blind fashion) either the ACE inhibitor or the placebo once daily for a week and, in the middle of that week, would undergo a second 24-hour blood-pressure monitoring.

We hypothesize that a positive placebo effect will occur: That is, in approximately one-third of those randomized to the placebo groups, blood pressure during therapy will be lower than baseline. We also hypothesize that reduction in blood pressure will be greater in the "matched" as compared to the "mismatched" groups. We are especially interested in seeing if the relative contributions of these two factors can be measured, in particular, whether the blood-pressure reduction in the placebo/match group might actually turn out to be greater than that for the active drug/mismatch group, as the meaning model might predict. The data analysis will also allow us to focus on specific correlates of blood-pressure (e.g., if blood pressure drops in the placebo subjects while they are awake but not during sleep, or when they are calm but not when they are angry).

It might appear at this point that the qualitative research approach has been totally abandoned in favor of quantitative data. However, a valuable qualitative component can easily be added to the design just described. This would entail conducting a second open-ended interview within a week or two after the completion of the therapy week, in which subjects would be asked to describe their thoughts about the medication and how it had worked on their blood pressure during the week of treatment. These subjective reports could then be compared with the subjects' group assignment and the actual blood-pressure readings. For instance, did those viewing the "match" videotapes report greater confidence that the drug was working? Did those viewing the "mismatch" videotapes report an increased incidence of side effects thought to be due to the medication? Since these interviews would be open-ended, it would not be possible to construct in advance a detailed list of experimental questions that might arise.

To add yet another wrinkle, there is the possibility of adding a further quantitative dimension to the study. Several possible biochemical mediators appear to be good candidates for the psychosomatic "link" in placebo reactions: catecholamines, endorphins, and immunoglobulins in particular (McClelland & Kirshnit, 1987). Previous laboratory work has suggested that viewing a film that has special meaning for the subject may produce measurable short-term changes in serum, urine or salivary concentrations of these substances (Brody, 1986). Accordingly, serum or urine samples could be collected for assay from our subjects before and after videotape viewings, and also during the week of therapy. As catecholamines may be most directly linked to blood pressure, it would be particularly interesting to see whether for instance, the levels of these substances dropped after viewings of the "match" but rose after the "mismatch" videotape, and whether these changes persisted later in the week.

Conclusion

I would imagine at this point that the advocate of qualitative research in primary care might be quite distressed with this example I have presented, since it employs many of the methods and approaches of the more usual quantitative paradigm. I would defend my choice by claiming that the case contains several essential features of the qualitative approach.

First, part of the reason I described the evolution of the study design in narrative form was to indicate that in important ways, the qualitative aspects of the research came first and the quantitative elements then came along for the ride. The turn toward what would appear to be objectively measurable was not an abandonment of the qualitative approach; rather, at a certain point in the development of the qualitative ideas and analysis, it seemed essential that the theory be "brought down to earth" in a particular way. That is, the theory had to be expressed in terms that made reference to specific sorts of bodily changes (as well as other terms that referred to an individual's thoughts and emotions, and the worldviews of various cultures). Therefore an essential way of refining and testing the theory would be to relate it back to observable and measurable bodily changes. Only in that way could the investigator be sure that the practical implications of the theory were as the theory claimed them to be; in short, that the theory was valid.

A closely related point involves the question of the "trust-worthiness" of qualitative or naturalistic research methods. Here I will again refer to Kuzel's (1986) review, which is based in this case on the prior work of Guba (1981). Any scientific work must meet the possible criticism that it is failing truly to describe the phenomena studied, or else that it is inapplicable to phenomena that occur elsewhere. Quantitative research usually meets these criticisms by employing methods such as control, randomization, and probabilistic sampling. Guba (as related by Kuzel) notes that qualitative research responds to them by employing methods such as triangulation and thick description. Now, in the case of ethnographic research, one may use these two methods in a strictly qualitative fashion. That is, in noting how the same phenomenon may be observed from several different viewpoints, all viewpoints considered will employ a qualitative description; and in describing a phenomenon with suitable "thickness" so that its historical and cultural context are accurately recorded, one will again use a qualitative approach for all aspects of the description.

However, there is no clear reason why triangulation might not entail the viewing of the same phenomenon from multiple view-points, some of which may be described qualitatively and some quantitatively. And there is no clear reason why a "thick descrip-tion" could not be seen to be in accordance with a systems hierarchy like Engel's (1977) biopsychosocial model, in which "thickness" comes precisely from involving levels of explanation that employ quantitative as well as qualitative approaches in a coordinated fashion. From the standpoint of primary care medi-cine, which must in practice coordinate both sorts of data and theories, crossing between the two research paradigms in the course of triangulation and thick description would appear to be a strength, not a sign of inconsistency. It is with this sense of complementarity in mind that I assert that the conjoint employ-ment of qualitative and quantitative methods in the research design described above counts as a positive example of adhering to the trustworthiness criteria of qualitative research, and also enhances the likelihood that the results will be illustrative of and applicable to primary care medical practice.

References

Adler, H. M., & Hammett, V. B. O. (1973). The doctor-patient relationship revisited: An analysis of the placebo effect. *Annals of Internal Medicine, 78,* 595-598.

Bass, M. J., Buck, C., Turner, L., Dickie, G., Pratt, G., & Robinson, H. C. (1983). The physician's actions and the outcome of illness. *Journal of Family Practice, 23,* 43-47.

Brody, H. (1980). *Placebos and the philosophy of medicine.* Chicago: University of Chicago Press.

Brody, H. (1986). The placebo response. *Drug Therapy, 16*(7), 106-131.

Brody, H. (1987). *Stories of sickness.* New Haven: Yale University Press.

Bruner, J. (1986). *Actual minds, possible worlds.* Cambridge, MA: Harvard University Press.

Cassell, E. J. (1976). *The healer's art: A new approach to the doctor-patient relationship.* Philadelphia: J. B. Lippincott.

Egbert, L. D., Battit, G. E., Welch, C. E., & Bartlett, M. K. (1964). Reduction in postoperative pain by encouragement and instruction of patients. *New England Journal of Medicine, 270,* 825-827.

Engel, G. L. (1977). The need for a new medical model: A challenge for biomedicine. *Science, 196,* 129-136.

Engel, G. L. (1988). How much longer must medicine's science be bound by a seventeenth century world view? In: K. L. White (Ed.), *The task of medicine: Dialogue at Wickenburg.* Menlo Park, CA: The Kaiser Family Foundation.

Greenfield, S., Kaplan, S., & Ware, J. E. (1985). Expanding patient involvement in care. *Annals of Internal Medicine, 102,* 520-528.

Guba, E. G. (1981). Criteria for assessing the trustworthiness of naturalistic inquires. *Education, Communication and Technology Journal, 29,* 75-91.

Headache Study Group of The University of Western Ontario, The. (1986). Predictors of outcome in headache patients presenting to family physicians—a one year prospective study. *Headache, 26,* 285-294.

Helman, C. G. (1981). "Tonic," "fuel" and "food": Social and symbolic aspects of the long-term use of psychotropic drugs. *Social Sciences in Medicine, 15B,* 521-533.

Herbert, C. P. (1988). Figure and ground: Reframing the study of decision making in family practice. *Family Medicine, 20,* 319ff.

Jonsen, A. L., & Toulmin, S. M. (1988). *The abuse of casuistry.* Berkeley: University of California Press.

Kuzel, A. J. (1986). Naturalistic inquiry: An appropriate model for family medicine. *Family Medicine, 18,* 369-374.

McClelland, D. C., & Kirshnit, C. (1987). The effect of motivational arousal through films on salivary immunoglobulin A. *Psychology and Health, 2,* 31-52.

VanEgeren, L., & Madarasmi, S. (1988). A computer-assisted diary (CAD) for ambulatory blood pressure monitoring. *American Journal of Hypertension, 1* (Suppl.), 179-185.

10 Standards of Trustworthiness for Qualitative Studies in Primary Care

ANTON J. KUZEL
ROBERT C. LIKE

Introduction

Several family medicine researchers have called for incorporating qualitative approaches so that we may address new questions, or address old ones in different ways (Addison, 1989b; Burkett & Godkin, 1983; Candib, 1988; Galazka & Eckert, 1986; Kuzel, 1986; Like & Steiner, 1986; McWhinney, 1989; Rainsberry, 1986). These few published reviews are representative of a larger group of primary care researchers who wish to pursue problems best approached by qualitative methods.

Yet those of us interested in qualitative research face many obstacles, not the least of which is the skepticism of our more quantitatively oriented colleagues. Some of the criticism may be based on circular logic, for according to Brody (Chapter 9), "It is fairly easy to 'prove' that quantitative methods are a superior way of gaining knowledge about the world, as long as we agree beforehand by social convention that we will regard only those questions that can easily be answered by quantitative methods as questions worth asking." Quantitative methods will also appear superior if one insists on applying quantitative means of insuring reliability and validity to qualitative research. "But is it rigorous?" is often asked of qualitative inquiry by those who are more familiar with the methods and standards of traditional, quantitative research.

In qualitative research, the most important people to decide the answer to the question of rigor or goodness are the researcher and the respondent. In a larger context, the researcher's community colleagues, funding sources, editors, and the respondent's community must be considered.

Many authors in fields of human science have suggested approaches to the problem of criteria for qualitative research. Anthropologists have published guides to ethnographic inquiry (Agar, 1980; Bernard, 1988; Fetterman, 1989; Geertz, 1973; Spradley, 1979; Werner & Schoepfle, 1986): a "model" for qualitative research in the same way that the experiment is a model for traditional research. Many examples of qualitative inquiry and much discussion of its standards may also be found in literature from sociology (Becker, 1970; Glaser & Strauss, 1967; Guldner, 1972; Lofland & Lofland, 1983; McCall & Simmons, 1969) and education (Bogdan & Biklen, 1982; Goetz & LeCompte, 1984; Guba, 1981; Lincoln & Guba, 1985, 1986; Marshall & Rossman, 1989; Miles & Huberman, 1984; Patton, 1980; Predo & Feinberg, 1982; Smith, 1989; Smith & Heshusius, 1986). Within the health sciences, nursing has shown particular leadership in defining and applying qualitative models to its research agenda (Cobb & Hagemaste, 1987; Rosenthal, 1989).

In addition to these disciplines that inform our consideration of standards for qualitative research, we must also recognize that there are many different kinds of qualitative research that pertain to primary care, as Helman has elaborated in Chapter 8. There will be some differences in the way we judge a personal narrative (Brody, 1987) as compared to a cultural anthropology study of health beliefs (Helman, 1984). Yet another layer in the discussion is the existence of multiple "subtraditions" within the larger tradition of qualitative research, among them "post-positivist," "constructivist," and "critical theorist," each with its own ideas about standards for its brand of qualitative inquiry (Kuzel, in press; Smith, 1989).

Given this bewildering array of traditions and standards, how are we in primary care to choose our criteria for qualitative inquiry? Some values that can guide our deliberations include:

pragmatism (the system should be useful for studies that can answer the questions we want to ask), tradition (we should consider those models already established for doing qualitative research in nonmedical fields), consensus (the system should receive the support of significant numbers of researchers in primary care), and familiarity (it should look enough like the traditional approach to be tolerated by those raised in the traditional approach). One can view the process of deciding upon standards for qualitative research in family medicine as itself a sort of qualitative inquiry. Indeed, the values we suggest above are strikingly parallel to the features of good qualitative research recently suggested by Addison (1989a): "If an answer has been uncovered by an interpretive account we should find it plausible, it should fit other material that we are aware of, other people should find it convincing, and it should have the power to change practice. These are the four approaches to evaluation [of an interpretive account]." They also parallel those offered by Kuzel (in press):

> As we practice, we are guided by concerns that may well serve as guides for other kinds of qualitative research that we do: Do our understanding and our practice make sense to us and to our patients (are they both internally coherent and externally connected to our past experiences)? Is our practice useful for our patient (does it address the concerns or problems that we have agreed upon)? Is our practice ethical (as defined by both physician and patient)? Finally, an addition suggested by William Miller (personal communication): Is our practice moral (do we have at heart the betterment of our patients and our community)?

Before considering the application of these guides for evaluating qualitative inquiry, we must comment on another theme that has surfaced in discussions about research traditions in primary care—that *combining* both quantitative and qualitative approaches within the same research endeavor will result in a better, more complete understanding of the phenomenon under study. One of us (RCL) suggests that primary care research ideally should be an integrative enterprise employing both quantitative and qualitative research methods. Although numerous books and articles have been written contrasting the philosophical foundations, working assumptions, purposes, and strengths and weaknesses of these research traditions, one can defend that the two must be linked if primary care research is to produce clinically relevant results that have "truth value," applicability, consistency, and neutrality (Fielding & Fielding, 1986; Guba, 1981). Furthermore, Miles and Huberman (1984), citing Cook and Reichardt's work, note that "qualitative and quantitative approaches are not operationally (or paradigmatically) incompatible." They comment that the latter's analysis carefully debunks "the stereotypes that qualitative researchers must necessarily be phenomenological, naturalistic, subjective, inductive, and holistic, while quantitative researchers must necessarily be positivistic, obtrusive, objective, deductive and particularistic."

The other of us (AJK) (Kuzel, 1986) asserts that there is no problem with combining quantitative and qualitative methods within a single research project, as long as one is talking about methods and not models or paradigms. One can make this distinction because traditional research tends to use quantitative methods, and interpretive research tends to use qualitative methods. Neither tradition excludes the use of the other's preferred methodologies, however. Where some tension does exist is at the level of epistemology, or "how you know that you know." The basic assumptions of the two traditions are so different (e.g., objective versus subjective reality; a need to understand cause-and-effect versus a need to understand meaning) that they may inevitably be at odds with one another if the researcher tries to mix them at the level of epistemology. A researcher should clearly specify and do justice to the inquiry paradigm of choice for a given question. One may, in some cases, certainly ask the same question using both traditions separately, but coming up with the same answer may not represent anything more than coincidence. It doesn't necessarily make the answer any more valid. The quantitative answer has a trustworthiness as judged by the standards of quantitative inquiry, and the qualitative answer has a trustworthiness as judged by the standards of qualitative, naturalistic inquiry (Guba, 1981; Lincoln & Guba, 1985). Perhaps we should curb our natural zeal for eclecticism with a concern that we do justice to the research traditions we choose to use.

With this background understanding, we now wish to explicate some means whereby qualitative researchers may address "goodness criteria." We will look at some procedures suggested by Lincoln and Guba (1985) and by Glaser and Strauss (1967) because they are well respected authors in their respective fields of education and sociology, and because their systems seem to us to be pragmatic and familiar—they lend themselves to translation into primary care research. The four procedures we choose to highlight here include member checking (Guba, 1981), searching for disconfirming evidence (Glaser & Strauss, 1967), triangulation (Guba, 1981), and thick description (Geertz, 1973; Guba, 1981). The first three enhance the "truth value" of an inquiry, and the last fosters the "transfer" of research findings to other settings (Lincoln & Guba, 1985).

Member Checking

"Member checking" refers to the process of dialogue between researcher and respondent/patient. The patient provides information and concepts, which the researcher must then interpret, that is, make sense of from the researcher's point of view. This interpretation is then given back to the patient, with a view to checking if it still makes sense from the patient's point of view. Although, as originally proposed by Guba (1981), this procedure seemed to be largely one that insured an accurate representation of the respondent's perspective (an *emic* rather than an *etic* picture: Pelto & Pelto, 1978), it seems that the continuing involvement of both researcher and patient in the process leads to a shared understanding and is a developmental process for both. Addison (1989a, 1989b) refers to this as the "hermeneutic circle" of interpretive inquiry, while Spradley (1979) describes ethnographic research as learning from a culture rather than studying it—consistent with this characterization of member checking.

In order to clarify this concept as well as the other three listed above, we sought examples from the papers and proposals reported in other chapters of this volume; specifically, Brody's research proposal in Chapter 9 and the collection of papers assembled by Tudiver in Chapter 11. We acknowledge that this is somewhat presumptuous, since it may be that the investigators were not guided by any preordained standards for qualitative research, but rather by the "norms of social discourse," which Smith (1989) has suggested is the only defensible stance regarding criteria for qualitative inquiry. Alternatively, they may have been guided by standards other than those that we have chosen to highlight in this discussion. Additionally, these papers are reported in a condensed form, which limits our ability to make any inferences about their quality. With these caveats in mind, we will attempt to illustrate the four selected features of qualitative research.

Most of the studies did not specifically provide evidence that the researchers had checked their understanding with their patients/respondents. It is entirely possible that, during the interview process, interviewers may have restated, summarized, or paraphrased what they thought they had just heard from the respondent—any of these would be a form of member checking. The one example of apparent member checking is found in Manca's description of the means whereby she addressed the "credibility and reproducibility" of her study, in which she states that "interpretations were clarified with the subjects" she interviewed (Chapter 11).

We might also illustrate this concept by looking at Brody's proposal concerning the placebo effect in the treatment of hypertension (Chapter 9). Brody uses two major approaches. The first is to elicit the patient's beliefs about blood-pressure control, via a questionnaire developed by more extensive interviews with a subsample of patients. He then looks for a demonstration of efficacy (lowering of blood pressure) in order to infer a congruence and thereby an acceptance of an explanatory model. This second step, using experimental and control groups, is entirely consistent with the quantitative tradition, and one can argue that it is the appropriate approach, given the quantitative effect under scrutiny (the control of hypertension). Additional approaches might be used, however, which focus more explicitly on the meaning of the model for the patient.

If Brody were to shift his stance in this study toward a more qualitative approach, he could choose to set aside the theory he developed from a review of existing literature, and derive one through interviews and observations of the patients in his own practice. It is entirely possible that he might thereby come up with the same theory, yet its creation would be tied more closely to the thoughts and beliefs of his own patients (Glaser & Strauss, 1967). Alternatively, or in addition, even after deriving the three to five basic types of patient explanatory models regarding blood-pressure control, he could periodically choose a patient whose belief system he could learn about in more depth through discussion, and from whom he could elicit reactions to the videotape selected as best fitting that patient's belief system. This is an addition that Brody himself suggests in the last section of his proposal, and seems to us to illustrate well the notion of "member checking."

Member checking enhances the likelihood that the results of an inquiry will represent the point of view of the respondent/patient, and is resonant with the medical credo to "learn from our patients." It is also consistent with the practice of the best primary care physicians, who explicitly involve their patients with formulations of diagnoses and constructions of treatment plans (Kuzel, in press; Like & Zyzanski, 1986, 1987).

The following questions should be explicitly addressed when incorporating member checking into the design of a qualitative research study. How will members be chosen, and how many need to participate? Who will be responsible for doing the member checking? Where will it take place? Will it occur in a group setting, or with individuals on a one-on-one basis? How frequently will it take place, and during what phase(s) of the research undertaking? In what form will information be presented to members? Probably most important, how will potential influences (i.e., "biases" or "threats") be monitored for and taken into account in enhancing the "truth value" of the inquiry?

Textbooks on sociological research methods have reviewed the types of investigator, respondent, interpersonal, and contextual influences that can impact on the interviewing process (Denzin, 1978; Jahoda, Deutsch, & Cook, 1951; Webb, Campbell, Schwartz, & Sechrest, 1966). Most of these should also apply to member checking.

With regard to investigator influences, Miles and Huberman (1984) quote Wax in suggesting the need to guard against:

1. the holistic fallacy: interpreting events as more patterned and congruent than they really are, lopping off the many loose ends of which social life is made;
2. elite bias: overweighing data from articulate, well-informed, usually high-status informants and under-representing data from intractable, less articulate, lower-status ones;
3. going native: losing one's perspective or one's "bracketing" ability, being coopted into the perceptions and explanations of local informants.(p. 230)

In addition, the investigator will need to deal with his/her own personal counter-transferential beliefs, feelings, and behaviors during the research undertaking (Powdermaker, 1966; Stein, 1985).

With regard to respondents, Lincoln and Guba (1985) suggest that individuals may:

- be unfamiliar with, misunderstand, or not be able to understand the information presented,
- believe the information to be biased,
- perceive the information to be in conflict with his/her self-interest, or,
- have an alternative interpretation of the information. (p. 243)

McCracken (1988) notes that this may lead to "impression management, topic avoidance, deliberate distortion, minor misunderstanding, and outright incomprehension" (p. 39).

With regard to interpersonal influences, the potential effects of investigator-respondent, investigator-investigator, and respondent-respondent relationships need to be considered. For example, are there any gender, racial/ethnic, social class, or power issues that may impact on the dialogue between investigator and respondent? For investigators engaged in a multidisciplinary project, are the research abilities and contributions of participants equally valued and permitted to enter into the member checking process, or are some investigators "more equal" than others? And among respondents engaged in a group member checking activity, how might group dynamics (e.g., social desirability response sets, competition, conspiracy, anger, fear) shape the types of information and interpretations that are discussed (Lincoln & Guba, 1985, p. 315)?

Finally, the spatial and temporal context in which member checking occurs must be considered. Will the site (e.g., the respondent's home or place of work, a clinic or hospital, the investigator's office) potentially have an impact, and if so, how? Is there a previous history of research with the respondent? Was that experience positive or negative? Are there any current or future considerations that might influence the member checking process?

Member checking is a critical feature of what might be termed the collaborative or negotiated approach to scientific knowledge production. Rather than controlling for potential "biases" or "threats" solely through the use of traditional methodological devices (e.g., random sampling, random allocation, control groups, matching, and other statistical operations), the investigator enters into a dialogue with respondents to make these influences explicit, and to give members an additional opportunity to confirm, clarify, challenge, critique, or correct the researcher's construction of reality. Member checking is a form of "empowerment" that has recently been suggested by Lincoln and Guba (1985) to be crucial in establishing the "fairness" or "justice" of a naturalistic inquiry.

Searching for Disconfirming Evidence

Searching for disconfirming evidence is another way of assuring the reader of the "validity" of the conclusions of a qualitative study, and was suggested by Glaser and Strauss (1967) in *The Discovery of Grounded Theory*. As applied to qualitative inquiry, it is the process whereby the researcher challenges his or her developing understanding about the subject of study by deliberately looking for evidence that challenges his or her understanding. If the search fails to yield such evidence, the conclusions are relatively stronger and more convincing than if the researcher had never tried to "knock them down." In operation within a qualitative study, one might ask a respondent, "Who thinks very differently from you about this subject?" In the process of theory construction, if one finds that A and B seem to always go together, one would look very hard for examples of situations in which they did not go together, in order to obtain a more accurate understanding of the relationship of A with B.

Again, the brief descriptions of the papers in Chapter 11 do not provide evidence of this technique, with the exception of Manca's study in which she states that "incongruencies were sought after and carefully assessed." Turning again to Brody's proposal, he suggests that, through qualitative interviews with patients, one might develop three to five explanatory models of blood-pressure control, assigning subsequent patients to one of these model categories based on a structured interview. We feel the proposal could be strengthened (from a qualitative point of view) by looking explicitly for patients whose explanatory models of blood-pressure control are *not* well described in any of these categories. If any were found, the investigator could respond by modifying the conceptual framework of the original categories or by adding additional ones. If none were found, we as readers would be relatively more convinced that the original schema was a good characterization of the explanatory models of blood-pressure control for this particular group of patients.

"Negative case analysis," according to Lincoln and Guba (1985), "may be regarded as a 'process of revising hypotheses with hindsight.' " It requires the researcher to develop understandings and explanations that cover a greater range of circumstances within the boundaries of the particular study. Although it is tempting to view this process as a means whereby one might draw more convincing causal inferences about relationships between people or events, it is more consistent with the qualitative inquiry traditions to think of the search for disconfirming evidence as helping the researcher create better explanations.

Rosenblatt (1981) has suggested that in order to engage in negative case analysis (or what Campbell [1975] elsewhere has called "degrees of freedom analysis"), the investigator must

- have a "tolerance for theory failure and an openness to evidence that one has made errors, perhaps enormous errors,"
- receive "training in how to think," in order to see alternative interpretations and to think through their implications, and,

- develop "theoretical fluency," "a sense of the relativity of theory and method," and an awareness that "specific theories and methods are useful in some situations, harmful in others." (pp. 220-221)

The researcher also needs to address the following difficult questions: What constitutes a negative case (e.g., does an "outlier" represent a challenge to the hypothesis, a chance occurrence, or an error in the data)? Should one insist on zero exceptions to the hypothesis, or is this too demanding a criterion? How should one deal with negative cases that in fact represent "lies, fronts, and other deliberate or unconscious deceptions" (Lincoln & Guba, 1985, p. 312)? How and where should the search for negative cases take place? When should this search begin, and when should it end? Finally, given the potential for large amounts of data, what are the available time and resources for undertaking negative case analyses?

There are certainly no easy or definitive answers to these questions. Each investigator will likely need to find solutions specific to his or her own study. Perhaps the advice of Miles and Huberman (1984) is most helpful: "Check out alternative explanations early, but don't iterate forever" (p. 241).

In summary, Kidder (1981) writes:

[E]ven though inductive analysis violates the assumptions of statistical testing by forming hypotheses to fit the data rather than finding data to test hypotheses, the consequences are not so different. When qualitative research has abundant evidence, it rings true, the conclusions are obvious, and they may be either interesting or trivial. When qualitative research has sparse evidence, it is not persuasive, even though there are no negative cases. Abundant evidence in qualitative research results when one has made many observations and recorded many instances. This is the equivalent of having a large N. The larger the N, the more convincing the conclusion in either case. (p. 244)

We wish to point out, however, that powerful and persuasive arguments can sometimes be constructed by using a few well-chosen pieces of evidence.

Triangulation

We next consider a third technique to enhance the credibility of qualitative inquiry: triangulation. The origin of the term probably relates to the notion of radio triangulation, whereby a source is pinpointed by getting a fix on it from two different points, then determining its location by constructing a triangle and applying principles of geometry. The analogy in qualitative inquiry is that one wishes to obtain multiple perspectives on a phenomenon—to see it from different angles—in order to create a more complete understanding. Triangulation is most often thought of as referring to obtaining information from multiple sources. Denzin (1978), however, asserts that one may also employ multiple and different methods, investigators, and theories. (In Chapter 9, Brody seems to suggest that one may employ a triangulation of paradigms within a study; we will have some comment on this idea below.)

Multiple data sources for a qualitative inquiry might include "multiple copies of one type of source (such as interview respondents) or different sources of the same information (for example, verifying an interview respondent's recollections about what happened at a board meeting by consulting the official minutes of that meeting)" (Lincoln & Guba, 1985). Multiple methods might include unobtrusive means such as document analysis or nonparticipant observation (Webb et al., 1966) or more obtrusive techniques such as participant observation or surveys (Denzin, 1978). By using multiple investigators, one is not expecting corroboration of one investigator by another so as to demonstrate replicability and reliability. The notion is rather that a richer, more encompassing understanding will result from employing several interpreters who collaborate with one another (Lincoln & Guba, 1985).

Triangulation of theories refers to examining a body of empirical data from a variety of theoretical perspectives. An example drawn from primary care might be analyzing doctor-patient communication during everyday clinical encounters using structuralist/functionalist theory, symbolic interactionism, exchange theory, semiotics, phenomenology, or critical theory. Earlier in this volume, Brody asserts that "there is no clear reason why triangulation might not entail the viewing of the same phenomenon from multiple viewpoints, some of which may be described qualitatively and some quantitatively." We agree. It is entirely reasonable to measure a patient's blood pressure and express it as a number, whereas the patient's explanatory model of blood-pressure control is elicited by dialogue and is expressed as a series of words that have meaning for the patient, researcher, and reader. The former may be understood with theory from physiology, and the latter with theory from symbolic interactionism. However, since Brody is addressing two different, albeit related, phenomena—the patient's blood pressure and the patient's explanatory model of blood-pressure control—we don't believe that he is actually engaging in triangulation on the same phenomenon.

Triangulation of data sources was not apparent in any of the reported studies in Chapter 11. Although several investigations involved interviews and structured questionnaires, none sought information from people other than the respondents (who were, in each case, a relatively homogenous group), nor was documentary evidence (such as medical charts) examined.

Triangulation of methods is evident in Brown's study (Chapter 11) of the impact of developmental antecedents on the personal and professional well-being of female family physicians. She employed both semistructured interviews and projective testing to develop a more complete understanding of the intrapsychic characteristics of her respondents and the implications of those characteristics for professional development. We would note, however, that the theoretical orientation of the study seemed to be established prior to contact with the respondents and appeared to be unaffected by the investigation. The categories of analysis also seemed predetermined. The process of data production was more a solicitation of information than a dialogue between investigator and respondent. These features give the study a less responsive flavor, leading us to view it as employing a traditional inquiry paradigm despite the use of qualitative methods.

Triangulation of investigators may be found in the papers by Cushman et al., and Manca (Chapter 11). In all of these studies the analysis of the qualitative data is done by multiple investigators, leading to a consensual interpretation.

In Cushman et al.'s (Chapter 11) investigation, triangulation is also employed in data production in that the elicitation of genograms and Life-Space diagrams is done by multiple investigators; but, as the authors themselves point out, the process is not well documented and the investigators apparently do not dialogue with one another at this point in the study. Both of these features make data interpretation more difficult and do not lend any additional credibility to the study. If one employs multiple investigators in a qualitative study, it is important that they have regular and documented discussion with one another as the process of data-gathering and interpretation proceeds (Lincoln & Guba, 1985).

There are some limitations of triangulation, particularly as it involves theory and paradigm, that deserve attention. The argument against triangulation of theories is given by Lincoln and Guba (1985):

> What can it mean that certain facts can be consistent with two or more theories? In what sense can it be the case that facts can be given more weight if they are consistent with multiple theories? We have noted repeatedly the likelihood that facts are, in the first instance, theory-determined; they do not have an existence independent of the theory within whose framework they achieve coherence. If a given fact is "confirmable" within two theories, that finding may be more a function of the similarity of theories than of the empirical meaningfulness of the fact. Further, theories can be interrelated; many "facts" within Newtonian theory are also facts within relativity theory, for example, because, in one sense, Newtonian theory can be taken as a "special case" of relativity theory. But the fact is not more believable because it has meaning within both these theories than if it had meaning in only one of them. The use of multiple theories as a triangulation technique seems to us to be both epistemologically unsound and empirically empty.

This echoes the earlier contention that employing quantitative (traditional) and qualitative (interpretive) paradigms to address the same question in hopes of coming up with the same answer may be defensible only as a means of getting traditional members of the audience to more readily believe the qualitatively derived answer.

One of us (AJK) believes that since "science is culturally bound and historically limited" (Popkewitz, 1981), the traditional inquiry paradigm can be viewed as a special case of qualitative, constructivist inquiry in the same way that Newtonian theory is a special case of the theory of relativity. The quantitative, positivist paradigm (and even the paradigms of post-positivism and critical theory) may be thought of as culturally defined ways of knowing that are epistemologically more bounded, and therefore subsets of the more encompassing paradigm variously labeled as qualitative inquiry, naturalism, or constructivism. The argument that Lincoln and Guba have made against triangulation of theory therefore applies in the same way to triangulation of paradigm.

The other of us (RCL) completely agrees that "science is culturally bound and historically limited," but is unsure whether the quantitative model of research can be seen as simply representing a "special case" of the qualitative paradigm. Indeed, there are alternative quantitative schools of research (e.g., exploratory data analysis) that have raised similar caveats about traditional inquiry methods and suggested the need for skepticism and openness in working with and learning from data (Hartwig & Dearing, 1979). As such, he would argue that these two methods of inquiry are dialectically related and represent two different ways of constructed knowing. He would also agree with McCracken (1988) that while the distinctness of each inquiry paradigm must be honored, "future research must be coordinated and ecumenical" (p. 15).

Besides these somewhat abstract concerns, there are practical questions that must be answered when employing triangulation. Denzin (1978) points out that:

- there may be problems in "locating a common unit of observation against which various theories can be applied,"
- the use of multiple methods and observers raises the possibility of additional methods and observer bias,
- limited time and money may "make it impossible to employ multiple observers, multiple methods, and multiple data sources," and

- there may be "inaccessibility of critical data areas, types, or levels." (pp. 311-312)

Fielding and Fielding (1986) add to this list the following:

- the use of a variety of methods "can actually increase the possibility of error" (especially when "bias checking procedures" are not included),
- the focus on the completeness of data obscures the fact that "differences between types of data can be as illuminating as their points of coherence," and
- there is a need for "ground rules" in the selection of data sources, methods, and theories—this can help "transform eclecticism into 'syntheticism'." (pp. 31-34)

Thick Description

Finally we turn to the notion of "thick description," whereby the transferability of study findings may be enhanced (Guba, 1981; Lincoln & Guba, 1985). Originally coined by Geertz (1973), the term refers to a detailed description of the context and process of a qualitative investigation so as to allow the reader to consider whether the product of the inquiry—the interpretation of the data—may be relevant in another context. Presumably, this other context will have to be similar enough (at least in theoretically important ways) to the original context of inquiry if one hopes to achieve some transfer of findings.

Lincoln and Guba (1985) point out that "the question of what constitutes 'proper' thick description is, at this stage in the development of naturalist theory, still not completely resolved." They suggest, however, that it should include "a thorough description of the context or setting within which the inquiry took place and with which the inquiry was concerned . . . [and] a thorough description of the transactions or processes observed in that context that are relevant to the problem, evaluand, or policy option."

In order to generate "thick descriptions," qualitative researchers need to consider the following issues:

1. How will "contexts" and "the transactions or processes observed in these contexts" be defined?
2. What will be the boundaries of the description (i.e., what is figure and ground, using Gestalt therapy terms)?
3. What information about context or process is relevant (or irrelevant) for the purposes of the inquiry?
4. Are there any "varieties of sampling errors" (e.g., "population restriction," "population stability over time," "population stability over areas")? (Webb, Campbell, Schwartz, & Sechrest, 1966, p. 36)
5. Are there any "access to content" problems (e.g., "restriction to content," "stability of content over time," "stability of content over areas")? (Webb et al., 1985, p. 36) [We note that points (4) and (5) are driven by "sampling" concerns of traditional research and may not apply in exactly the same way to qualitative inquiry (Marshall & Rossman, 1989; Patton, 1980).]
6. How much information is needed for the final report (i.e., how "thick" or "thin" should the description be)?

The answers to these questions will help shape the nature of "the data base that makes transferability judgments possible on the part of potential appliers" (Lincoln & Guba, 1985, p. 316).

The notion of relevancy suggested by Lincoln and Guba is an important guide in deciding what features of context or process one should include in the final report of a qualitative investigation. The brevity of the reports in this volume precludes pointing to any actual examples, but a bit of speculation may illustrate the concept. For example, in Manca's description of the miscarriage experience, she states that her interviews "revealed the distress of the husband as described by the women." In deciding whether this notion of the husbands' distress and its part in their wives' miscarriage experience might transfer to another setting, it might be important to characterize the female respondents with respect to age, parity, length of marriage, etc. (assuming that these can be demonstrated to have some theoretical importance in understanding the miscarriage experience). One might also wish to have a better appreciation for the relationship between the women and their husbands before, during, and after the miscarriage, as well as the role that their relationships with other significant individuals (friends, family) may have played. If the particular sample selected by Manca drew mainly from nuclear families who were somewhat isolated, the significance of the relationship between husband and wife and the burdens placed upon it might be expected to be relatively greater than would be seen in extended family systems. On the other hand, it might be comparatively less important to report in any detail on contextual features (such as the economic base of the community or climatic conditions) if these had no apparent theoretical bearing in this particular study. (This does not, of course, preclude the potential importance of these factors in a different context.)

In Chapter 9 Brody has suggested an expansion of Geertz's (1973) original meaning for thick description. He asserts:

> There is no clear reason why a "thick description" could not be seen according to a systems hierarchy like Engel's biopsychosocial model, in which "thickness" comes precisely from involving levels of explanation which employ quantitative as well as qualitative approaches, in a coordinated fashion. From the standpoint of primary care medicine, which must in practice coordinate both sorts of data and theories, crossing between the two research paradigms in the course of . . . thick description would appear to be a strength, not a sign of inconsistency.

We interpret Brody's assertion to mean that theory building that allows one to explain events at many levels, using both quantitative and qualitative information, is a good thing. If this is accurate, then we agree with Brody. We would not see this practice as a "crossing between the two research paradigms" simply because of mixed methodology, however. To illustrate, if one is describing and explaining the biochemical basis for the control of blood pressure by a given medication, one may appropriately construct and support theories using the traditional model—it works when one is concerned with biochemical and physiological processes. It does not work very well if one seeks to interpret the meaning of the patient's explanatory model for control of blood pressure. The qualitative approach seems called for in that case. We therefore see different inquiry paradigms being appropriately applied to different research questions within the same study. The paradigms may happen to have some relationship within the context of the study, but they should remain clearly identified and separated from one another.

Conclusion

McWhinney (1989) predicts that "we in family medicine will continue to use the conventional method of natural science whenever it is appropriate; our greatest contribution to medicine, however, may be in leading the way to a new method . . ." We are grateful for the efforts of those we have cited in this review who have provided examples and guidance for us as we strive to do good qualitative primary care research.

References

Addison, R. B. (1989a). Evaluating an interpretive account. In M. J. Packer & R. B. Addison (Eds.), *Entering the circle: Hermeneutic inquiry in psychology*. Albany: State University of New York Press.

Addison, R. B. (1989b). Grounded interpretive research: An investigation of physician socialization. In M. J. Packer & R. B. Addison (Eds.), *Entering the circle: Hermeneutic inquiry in psychology*. Albany: State University of New York Press.

Agar, M. H. (1980). *The professional stranger: An informal introduction to ethnography*. Orlando, FL: Academic Press.

Becker, H. S. (1970). *Sociological work: Method and substance*. New York: Aldine.

Bernard, H. R. (1988). *Research methods in cultural anthropology*. Newbury Park, CA: Sage.

Bogdan, R. C., & Biklen, S. K. (1982). *Qualitative research for education: An introduction to theory and method*. Boston: Allyn & Bacon.

Brody, H. (1987). *Stories of sickness*. New Haven: Yale University Press.

Burkett, G. L., & Godkin, M. A. (1983). Qualitative research in family medicine. *Journal of Family Practice, 16*, 625-626.

Campbell, D. T. (1975). "Degrees of freedom" and the case study. *Comparative Political Studies, 8*, 178-183.

Candib, L. (1988). Ways of knowing in family medicine. *Family Medicine, 20*, 133-136.

Cobb, A. K., & Hagemaste, J. N. (1987). Ten criteria for evaluating qualitative research proposals. *Journal of Nursing Education, 26*(4), 138-143.

Denzin, N. K. (1978). *The research act: A theoretical introduction to sociological methods*. New York: McGraw-Hill.

Fetterman, D. M. (1989). *Ethnography: Step by step*. Newbury Park, CA: Sage.

Fielding, N. G., & Fielding, J. L. (1986). *Linking data*. Newbury Park, CA: Sage.

Galazka, S. S., & Eckert, J. K. (1986). Clinically applied anthropology: Concepts for the family physician. *Journal of Family Practice, 22*, 159-165.

Geertz, C. (1973). *The interpretation of cultures*. New York: Basic Books.

Glaser, B. G., & Strauss, A. L. (1967). *The discovery of grounded theory: Strategies for qualitative research*. New York: Aldine.

Goetz, J., & LeCompte, M. (1984). *Ethnography and qualitative design in educational research.* New York: Academic Press.

Guba, E. G. (1981). Criteria for assessing the trustworthiness of naturalistic inquiries. *Education, Communication and Technology Journal, 29,* 75-91.

Guldner, A. (1972). *The coming crisis of Western sociology.* New York: Basic Books.

Hartwig, F., & Dearing, B. E. (1979). *Exploratory data analysis.* Newbury Park, CA: Sage.

Helman, C. G. (1984). *Culture, health and illness: An introduction for health professionals.* Bristol: Wright.

Jahoda, M., Deutsch, M., & Cook, S. W. (Eds.). (1951). *Research methods in social relations. Part 2: Selected techniques.* New York: Dryden Press.

Kidder, L. H. (1981). Qualitative research and quasi-experimental frameworks. In M. B. Brewer & B. E. Collins (Eds.), *Scientific inquiry and the social sciences.* San Franscisco: Jossey-Bass.

Kuzel, A. J. (1986). Naturalistic inquiry: An appropriate model for family medicine. *Family Medicine, 18,* 369-374.

Kuzel, A. J. (in press). Stranger in a strange land . . . *Family Medicine.*

Like, R. C., & Steiner, R. P. (1986). Medical anthropology and the family physician. *Family Medicine, 18,* 87-92.

Like, R. C., & Zyzanski, S. J. (1986). Patient requests in family practice: A focal point for clinical negotiations. *Family Practice, 3,* 216-228.

Like, R. C., & Zyzanski, S. J. (1987). Patient satisfaction with the clinical encounter: Social psychological determinants. *Social Sciences and Medicine, 24,* 351-357.

Lincoln, Y. S., & Guba, E. G. (1985). *Naturalistic inquiry.* Newbury Park, CA: Sage.

Lincoln, Y. S., & Guba, E. G. (1986). But is it rigorous? Trustworthiness and authenticity in naturalistic evaluation. In D. D. Williams (Ed.), *Naturalistic evaluation. New Directions for Program Evaluation, 90.* San Francisco: Jossey-Bass.

Lofland, J., & Lofland, L. (1983). *Analyzing social settings.* Belmont, CA: Wadsworth.

Marshall, C., & Rossman, G. B. (1989). *Designing qualitative research.* Newbury Park, CA: Sage.

McCall, G. J., & Simmons, J. L. (Eds.). (1969). *Issues in participant observation.* Redding, MA: Addison-Wesley.

McCracken, G. (1988). *The long interview.* Newbury Park, CA: Sage.

McWhinney, I. (1989). An acquaintance with particulars . . . *Family Medicine, 21,* 296-298.

Miles, M. S., & Huberman, A. M. (1984). *Qualitative data analysis: A sourcebook of new methods.* Newbury Park, CA: Sage.

Patton, M. (1990). *Qualitative evaluation and research methods.* Newbury Park, CA: Sage.

Pelto, P. J., & Pelto, C. H. (1978). *Anthropological research: The structure of inquiry* (2nd ed.). Cambridge, UK: Cambridge University Press.

Popkewitz, T. S. (1981). The study of schooling: Paradigms and field-based methodologies in educational research and evaluation. In T. S. Popkewitz & T. Tabachnik (Eds.), *The study of schooling: Paradigms and field-based methodologies in educational research and evaluation.* New York: Praeger.

Powdermaker, H. (1966). *Stranger and friend: The way of an anthropologist.* New York: W. W. Norton.

Predo, E., & Feinberg, W. (1982). *Knowledge and values in educational research.* Philadelphia: Temple University Press.

Rainsberry, R. P. (1986). Values, paradigms and research in family medicine. *Family Practice, 3,* 209-215.

Rosenblatt, P. C. (1981). Ethnographic case studies. In M. B. Brewer & B. E. Collins (Eds.), *Scientific inquiry and the social sciences.* San Franscisco: Jossey-Bass.

Rosenthal, T. T. (1989). Using ethnography to study nursing education. *Western Journal of Nursing Research,* 115-127.

Smith, J. K. (1989, March). *Alternative research paradigms and the problem of criteria.* Paper presented at the International Conference on Alternative Paradigms for Inquiry, San Francisco.

Smith, J. K., & Heshusius, L. (1986). Closing down the conversation: The end of the quantitative-qualitative debate among educational inquirers. *Educational Researcher, 15,* 4-12.

Spradley, J. P. (1979). *The ethnographic interview.* New York: Holt, Reinhart & Winston.

Stein, H. (1985). *The psychodynamics of medical practice.* Berkeley: University of California Press.

Webb, E. J., Campbell, D. T., Schwartz, R. D., & Sechrest, L. (1966).*Unobtrusive measures: Nonreactive research in the social sciences.* Chicago: Rand-McNally.

Werner, 0., & Schoepfle, M. (1986). *Systematic fieldwork.* Newbury Park, CA: Sage.

11 Combining Quantitative and Qualitative Methodologies in Primary Care: Some Examples

FRED TUDIVER
ROBERT A. CUSHMAN
BENJAMIN F. CRABTREE
WILLIAM L. MILLER
DONNA PATRICIA MANCA
JUDITH BELLE BROWN

Introduction (Tudiver)

Most research on primary medical care has depended on traditional quantitative methodologies for assessing interventions (Kleinbaum, Kupper, & Morgenstern, 1982). These techniques originated in biostatistics and epidemiology, both of which have their origins in agriculture. The quantitative paradigm relies on numeric data, collected through methods such as randomized trials, case-controlled studies, and observation. Statistics are then applied to these data to determine standardized ways of demonstrating change resulting from interventions.

In the past few years some primary medical care researchers have begun to employ qualitative methods to assess interventions (Kuzel, 1986; Like & Steiner, 1986; Prince-Embury, 1984). Using techniques that mostly derive from anthropology, this paradigm entails collecting observational and descriptive data through methods such as participant observation, case studies, and ethnography.

Each of these two approaches has major strengths and weaknesses. A quantitative study starts with a hypothesis, which it then tries to prove or refute. The methods are deductive, precise, objective, readily analyzed by computers, and often easily reproduced in other settings. However, they have also been described as rigid, closed, reductionist, and limited or "thin" in what they can explain about *how* and *why* interventions work.

In contrast, qualitative methods have been described as inductive, open, and rich, as they can often help explain how and why interventions work by elaborating on the *meaning* of the findings. Here, researchers start with observations, then lead up to theory and hypotheses: the opposite direction of the quantitative approach. However, the methods can be very labor-intensive, often requiring highly trained observers, and the data can be difficult to analyze and reproduce.

Recently several writers have discussed the integration of the two methods to study the same population. With this combined approach, an intervention can be assessed quantitatively, while the addition of qualitative data can help explain what Howard Brody calls the "meaning" of the findings (Chapter 9). Strange and Zyzanski's recent paper (1989) looks at some applications for combining the two methods, including:

- using both methods to cross-validate each other. In two studies, one on the functioning of the elderly (Ford et al., 1988) and the other on the predictability of a measure used in patients in a medical ICU (Kruse, Thill-Baharozian, & Carlson, 1988), informal qualitative measures were successfully used to cross-validate standard quantitative measures (the OARS and the APACHE II, respectively).

- combining quantitative and qualitative measures to determine potential biases (e.g., confounding, selection, or information biases). For example, in a study of diarrheal diseases in Central America, Scrimshaw and Hurtado (1988) reduced information bias by using ethnographic methods to compare subjects' terms for disease with standard medical terms.

- the two methods can be used concurrently to add "richness" or "thickness" to the quantitative study results. Dr. Brody's chapter (9) has an example of this technique.
- adding qualitative data in traditional randomized controlled trials to determine the generalizability of the findings. Stange and Zyzanski (1989) caution that such trials may entail unusually highly motivated subjects in artificial settings and recommend using case histories and key informant interviews to describe the study environment and its effect on subjects.

There are few examples in the literature of combining quantitative and qualitative methods in the primary care setting. In this chapter we present three cases of well-designed studies that have done so.

Cushman, Crabtree, and Miller tackle the difficult-to-define, difficult-to-measure, and context-sensitive concept of social support in the elderly, by using traditional quantitative measures along with qualitatively based tools (life-space diagrams and genograms). Their preliminary analyses demonstrate several of the uses of the benefits noted above: cross-validation of different methods, minimizing biases (especially information bias), and adding richness and thickness to their findings.

Manca's paper looks at the relationship between post-miscarriage distress and social support. Using both quantitative and qualitative analyses, she obtains a deeper understanding of the issues, new information that would not have been captured with either method used alone, and different ways of understanding (for example, she analyzes interviews through three perspectives—that of a physician, a woman, and a visitor from another society).

Brown's paper explores the developmental antecedents affecting the personal and professional well-being of a group of female family physicians. She uses quantitative measures in one phase of her study, and qualitative methods in the other to specifically identify some of these antecedents. As with Manca's, this study adds richness and data that would be difficult to obtain had it been confined to quantitative methods.

Life-Space Diagrams and Genograms as Measures of Social Support in the Elderly (Cushman, Crabtree, and Miller)

INTRODUCTION

The concept of "social support" is difficult to define and measure, although many instruments developed over the years have cumulatively striven to clarify it (O'Reilly, 1988; Orth-Gomer & Unden, 1987). Most of these have been *quantitative*, composed of lists of multiple-choice or true-false questions pertinent to researchers' specific interests (which are often poorly generalizable), and *research-oriented* (not readily adaptable for clinical use with individuals).

Therefore, when we set out to study the impact of social/environmental factors on nursing home admissions of the elderly, we sought both quantitative structural data and contextual information that might be analyzed by qualitative text analysis and/or by simple interpretive viewing. Our method was to collect Life-Space diagrams ·(Blake, 1988) and genograms (McGoldrick & Gerson, 1986) on individual subjects and compare their results against those obtained from some standardized questionnaires.

METHODS

A pilot study involved interviews with eight recently admitted elderly residents of a skilled nursing facility. An interviewer constructed a genogram on each respondent, and a Life-Space diagram was drawn either by the subject or the interviewer, depending on the capabilities of the former (see Results below). In addition, a series of four questionnaires was administered: the Mini-Duke Assessment of Functional Health Status (Blake & Vandiver, 1986), an adaptation of the Social Readjustment Rating Scale (SRRS) (Holmes & Rahe, 1967), a family support scale developed by researchers at Case Western Reserve University (Reeb, Graham, Zyzanski, & Kitson, 1987), and the FACES III (Olson, 1986).

Based on experiences gained from the pilot, for the main study some modifications were made to the Life-Space diagram and a shorter questionnaire packet was used, consisting of the Mini-

Mental Status Exam (MMSE) (Folstein, Folstein, & McHugh, 1975), the modified SRRS, and an instrument developed by Seeman and Berkman (1988) for the assessment of social support in the elderly. Six physicians, attending the geriatric research fellowship at the Travellers Center on Aging, conducted the interviews. A total of 17 elderly subjects were interviewed: 14 from four different nursing homes and three who lived independently in the community. All subjects were more than 65 years of age, had been discharged from a hospitalization within eight weeks, and were deemed mentally competent (a total score of at least 23 on the MMSE was required prior to further questioning).

For each individual, the questionnaire data were coded and scored, then compared with a *quantitative* analysis of the Life-Space diagrams and genograms, which was generated by counting the various types of individuals, qualities of relationships, and/or events indicated on them. Given the lack of identification of different *types* of individuals on the Life-Space diagram, we used color-coding or shape-coding to differentiate family, friends, and institutions, which proved to be helpful.

A *qualitative* analysis of each Life-Space diagram/genogram pair entailed its being interpreted independently by two of the authors. A verbal description and interpretation were dictated and later transcribed into a text format that included interpretations of the Life-Space diagram and genogram separately, as well as an overall impression. Using an a priori codebook, text from a subject was independently coded by each of the three authors and compared, using the methodology described by Miles and Huberman (1984). Marginal notes were used to revise the codebook, and the same text was again coded and checked for consistency. The codebook was then further revised, using data from another individual, and so on until it could be used satisfactorily.

RESULTS

During the pilot phase it quickly became clear that the Life-Space diagram could not be completed independently as a self-report instrument, because problems of visual acuity and manual dexterity prevented most of these elderly subjects from reading the instructions and/or handling a pencil to draw the symbols themselves. However, most were willing and able to understand

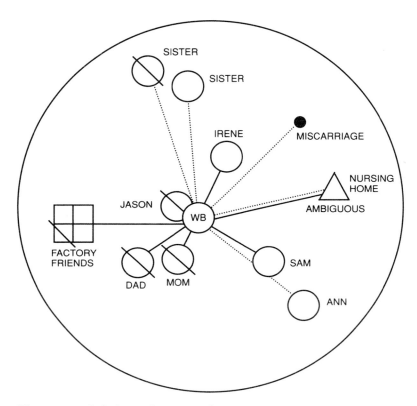

Figure 11.1. Life-Space Diagram of Respondent #302

the directions when given verbally and direct the interviewer as to where to draw the symbols. This interactive format was then adopted as the standard mode (see Figures 11.1 and 11.2 for examples).

Upon debriefing, interviewers noted that both they and the subjects seemed to find the more open, conversational format of the genogram more enjoyable than the tedious multiple questions of the survey questionnaires. The time taken to administer the combination of genogram and Life-Space diagram was

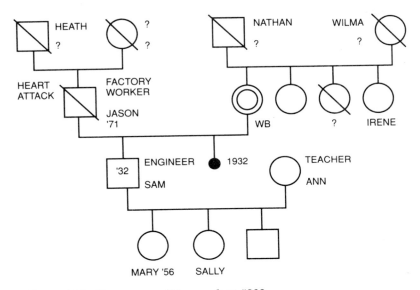

Figure 11.2. Genogram of Respondent #302

approximately equal to that taken for the questionnaires (in the pilot study the larger questionnaire packet had been too time-consuming, which motivated this change).

The comparison of quantitative information collected by the Life-Space/genogram combination and by the Seeman/Berkman Social Support Questionnaire was interesting. The basic quantitative data about numbers of family members were fairly consistent, except that the questionnaire neglected children-in-law and the deceased, who both appeared frequently as significant individuals on the Life-Space diagrams. Also, the diagrams gave a more in-depth picture of the friends network than did the single designation on the Seeman/Berkman and had the advantage of displaying family, friends, and institutions on the same scale regarding closeness. What the diagrams lacked quantitatively were specific data related to the frequency of communication, the identity of any persons helping with daily tasks, and the subjects' satisfaction with three items: childrens' visits, instrumental support provided, and emotional support received.

The interviewers were inconsistent in their recording of data on the genograms, especially regarding geographic location of family, occupations, medical conditions, and dates of key events in the lives of the individuals identified on the genograms. Another inconsistency was use of the wrong symbols on the Life-Space diagrams; these errors were usually detected when the companion genograms were evaluated.

The qualitative interpretation of the Life-Space/genograms is still in progress as of this publication, since the coding step is the most time-consuming. (An early example of the codebook is illustrated in Table 11.1.) Interestingly, the different coders made very similar categorizations and margin notes, so the codebook evolution progressed smoothly. Preliminary findings from this process indicate that a much richer depiction of the individual and his or her context is achieved. Common themes include deaths, grief, coping strategies, sibling connections, and occupational friend connections. These will be explored further as more cases are analyzed.

DISCUSSION AND FUTURE DIRECTIONS

Children-in-law and "the deceased" appeared frequently on the Life-Space diagrams of these elderly subjects, so they would appear to be an important source of social and emotional support not measured on existing structured social support questionnaires. Ascertaining the role that children-in-law play in comparison with other family and with nonfamilial friends in the emotional and instrumental support of the elderly warrants further research. A history of prior support with deceased persons who *had* been close may still play an active role in an individual's current sense of being "supported"; this may well be more important for the elderly than for other age groups.

One plan for further analysis of these instruments is the inclusion of literal primary data, such as tape-recordings of the interviews, which could then be subjected to text analysis and coding. The goals of this would be to ascertain (a) how well the interviewers record the data related to them, and (b) how well the

Table 11.1 Code Manual for Life-Space/Genogram Text

Activities	ACT
ACT: Car/transportation	ACT-CAR
ACT: Civic Groups	ACT-CIVIC
ACT: Family Gatherings/reunions	ACT-FAM
ACT: Hobbies/Avocation	ACT-HOB
ACT: Music	ACT-MUSIC
ACT: Sports	ACT-SPORTS

Church	CH
CH: Clergy	CH-CLERGY
CH: Heaver	CH-HEAVEN
CH: Groups	CH-GROUPS

Communication	COMM
COMM: Good	COMM-G
COMM: Fair	COMM-F
COMM: Poor	COMM-P

Coping Style	COPE
COPE: Denial	COPE-DENIAL

Death	DEATH
DEATH: Afterlife	DEATH-AFTER
DEATH: Child	DEATH-CHILD
DEATH: Funeral	DEATH-FUNERAL
DEATH: Grave	DEATH-GRAVE
DEATH: Grief	DEATH-GRIEF
DEATH: Miscarriage	DEATH-MISC
DEATH:Widowed	DEATH-WIDOW

Dependency	DEPEND
DEPEND: Caregiver—Family	DEPEND-FAM
DEPEND: Caregiver—Non-Family	DEPEND-NONFAM
DEPEND: Independence	DEPEND-IND

Diagram	DIAG
DIAG: Focus-Female Perdominance	DIAG-FOCUS/FEMALE
DIAG: Focus-Male Perdominance	DIAG-FOCUS/MALE
DIAG: Image, Picture	DIAG-IMAGE

investigators' interpretive descriptions fit with the subjects' own perspectives (i.e., to serve as a "reference" for both triangulation and reflexivity).

The Life-Space diagram could easily be adapted in future studies to include specifics such as communication frequency and identification of the providers of instrumental support. Addressing subjects' *satisfaction* with their current contact/communication/support would be more complex, but may be possible. Another possible adaptation would be the placement of concentric rings on the Life-Space circle, to facilitate determination of relative closeness to various individuals.

In summary, the potential usefulness of the combined Life-Space diagram and genogram as both a research tool and as a clinical instrument looks promising. In particular, including both quantitative and qualitative analyses of this combination is not only feasible, but at a depth that is not attainable by either method alone.

Study of Miscarriage Through Qualitative and Quantitative Methods (Manca)

INTRODUCTION

After observing reactions in women who miscarried, I sought a research method that would provide a better understanding of this experience and test the hypothesis that high distress is related to less support. Qualitative or quantitative methods alone would not satisfy my curiosity; therefore, I did a pilot study combining the two approaches. This paper illustrates the similarities and differences of these two methods, as they applied here, and demonstrates how they can complement each other.

PURPOSE

The type of question determines the approach to research. Qualitative methods apply when the question is broad with specific aims, such as what is asked to understand a patient's illness. With quantitative methods the question is focused and requires specific answers, such as what is asked to diagnose a disease or determine its etiology. The present study asked broad questions with specific aims to describe the emotional reaction following miscarriage and identify factors perceived to relieve or aggravate the distress. The specific hypotheses tested were that high support, from a) family and friends and b) from the physician, would be related to less distress four and 12 weeks after miscarriage.

METHODS

Participating physicians gave a letter explaining the study to patients who had miscarried, and those who agreed to participate then contacted me to arrange face-to-face interviews four and 12 weeks after the event. Each interview consisted of a structured (quantitative) and a semistructured (qualitative) segment. The structured segment had specific questions and measurements: Here, demographic data were obtained, distress and support quantified, inclusion and exclusion criteria evaluated, and important factors assessed. During the semistructured segment, descriptions of the miscarriage experience and what helped or aggravated it were obtained and assessed, using a qualitative methodology (Chenitz & Swanson, 1986; Glaser & Strauss, 1967; Gorden, 1980; Schatzman & Strauss, 1973; Strauss, 1987).

The questionnaires used to quantify distress and support included the 12-item General Health Questionnaire (GHQ), which measured general emotional health (Goldberg, 1972; Goldberg & Blackwell, 1970; Goldberg & Hillier, 1979); the 15-item Impact of Event Scale (IES), which quantified distress specific to miscarriage (Horowitz, Wilner, & Alverez, 1979; Kaltreider, Wallace, & Horowitz, 1979; Tennen & Herzberger, 1985; Zilberg, Weiss, & Horowitz, 1982); the Provisions of Social Relations Scale (PSR), which measured support from family and friends (Turner, 1983; Turner, Frankel, & Levin, 1983); and the Medical Interview Satisfaction Scale (MISS), which assessed physician support (Stiles, 1978; Stiles, Putnam, James, & Wolf, 1979; Wolf, Putnam, James, & Stiles, 1978). These instruments all have proven validity and reliability.

A number of important variables were also assessed: partner support (Nuttal, 1988), age, socioeconomic status of the household (Blishen & McRoberts, 1971), time to conceive, pain with the miscarriage (Melzack & Torgerson, 1971), length of warning symptoms, gestation at the time of miscarriage, physician variables, level of education, children, prior miscarriage, planned pregnancy, awareness that miscarriage can happen, and difficulty becoming pregnant prior to the miscarriage.

For the semistructured segment, following a pilot on four volunteers this question was developed: "I will now turn to the miscarriage itself. I would like to better understand what helped you or made things more difficult. Could you tell me your story from just before the pregnancy to now?" Rich descriptions of the experience were thereby obtained. Once the woman finished her story, I then asked: "What helped or made things more difficult? What could have been done differently?"

These interviews were tape-recorded, and I transcribed the first five myself. It took me eight hours to transcribe one hour of interview, but by doing this myself, I became aware of meanings I would have missed otherwise. Certain meaningful words were used that I had not noticed when just listening to the recordings— for example, "The doctors were there and said, 'Your wife is losing *your* child' " (italics added).

I listened to each interview a minimum of three times, from the perspectives of a physician, a woman, and a visitor from another society, to obtain information from the data that would not have been observed from one perspective. When I listened as a woman, I heard things I had missed when I approached the data as a physician. For example, I became more aware of women's roles and the issues of producing a son. The most difficult perspective to attain was that of another society. To do this I read about other cultures and their rituals. This helped me to notice how death was viewed as unclean when we describe a D&C as "cleaning" the womb.

As I developed a greater understanding, I became more able to code and categorize the information. For example, the category of "painful reminders" emerged as the women described things that reminded them of the miscarriage and their loss. Coded transcripts from two interviews were assessed by another physician to clarify the interpretation behind the words.

I took field notes, on descriptions of what I observed, and derived my theories or interpretations from these observations. In addition, during the first interview with each subject, I took methodological notes that served as reminders of information required to complete the second interview. By reviewing these notes and listening to tapes of the earlier interview, I knew which areas required further clarification. At the second interview my questions included: "What has happened since we last spoke? . . . Any further comments?" After the woman completed her story I then clarified unclear areas.

The qualitative data were continuously analyzed deductively and inductively, looking at similarities and differences and attempting to detect patterns as they emerged. Linkages between categories were determined, and an understanding of the emotional reaction to miscarriage, including relieving and aggravating factors, was sought out.

To improve credibility and reproducibility, different techniques were used with each method. With the quantitative method the interviews were standardized: Questions were asked in a specific order and in a specific way, and instruments with proven reliability and validity were used. With the qualitative method, reliability and validity were addressed by:

- Time: as much as six hours was spent with one subject.
- Review and re-review: interviews were listened to a minimum of three times, and transcripts were read many times.
- Different perspectives: interviews were listened to from various perspectives by the researcher, and another physician, who had an interest in anthropology, read a few of the transcripts and provided insights.
- Multiple sources of information: these were not practical here, but the literature supported some of the findings (Swanson-Kauffman, 1983).
- Peer review: coded transcripts were assessed by another physician to check interpretations.
- Clarification: interpretations were clarified with the subjects.
- Incongruencies: any were sought after and carefully assessed.

Sample size is another aspect that is in part determined by the methodology used. With a quantitative study the questions are brief and specific, so a larger number of subjects can be assessed. Also, a quantitative study must be powerful enough to detect an association when one exists. Based on this, a sample size of 20 was aimed for, since a smaller sample would have increased the likelihood of missing a true association.

In contrast, qualitative methods take more time, resulting in a greater depth of information from a smaller number of subjects. Here, a sample size of 10 was felt to be appropriate. The quality of the informant is important here: One woman who can clearly describe her experience is better than several who cannot articulate. Another factor is the saturation point of the researcher; in my case this occurred by approximately the twelfth interview, and I could find no new information after this time.

RESULTS

The combination of these two methods added a deeper understanding to the observations made: The quantitative data enabled specific questions to be answered, while the qualitative descriptions provided a better understanding of the factors under study. For example, the meaning of the pregnancy could be quantified to compare it to the distress measured, which would not have been possible with either method alone.

The open approach of the qualitative method provided new information and insights. For instance, it revealed the distress of the husbands as described by the women and illuminated the important role played by the physicians—observations that were not captured by the quantitative instruments used to measure the support from husband and physician.

The qualitative and quantitative aspects of the research may have interfered with one another. The semistructured interview could have acted as a catharsis, lowering the level of distress, especially for those women without support; or it may have distanced the women enough from a sensitive subject to enable them to do a lengthy structured interview in a matter-of-fact style.

DISCUSSION

Both quantitative and qualitative methods are important; however, medical research has tended to focus on the former. Quantitative research values information that can be generalized to a broad group, but this is not always helpful when treating Patient X, whose unique illness is not explained by the generalizations. Qualitative research seeks *understanding*: By understanding Patient X and his or her illness in depth, we may come to better understand others. There may be both similarities and differences to other patients, and patterns may unfold. For findings to be meaningful, we must develop specific questions that are appropriate for quantitative analysis and that are also close to the subject under study. Maybe quantitative and qualitative research simply represent different ways of knowing. As with a rose, with its aroma and its rich color, can we not better understand the rose by both seeing and smelling?

The Impact of Developmental Antecedents on the Personal and Professional Well-being of Female Family Physicians (Brown)

INTRODUCTION

This study explores developmental antecedents affecting the personal and professional well-being of a group of female family physicians. High functioning was defined as high self-esteem, an absence of depression or anxiety, a capacity to manage life stressors, work satisfaction, and a strong social support system. It was proposed that exhibition of these factors would be associated with greater evidence of identity of self as separate from others. Levels of identity formation were defined from a developmental perspective that identifies the achievement of psychological separation from primary objects as the major early life task. The prediction was that women who enter male-dominated high-stress professions such as medicine are more vulnerable to psychological problems if this self-other identify formation has been only partially achieved.

PHASE I

Methodology

The study consisted of two phases. In Phase I, a mailing went out to all practicing female family physicians in the area of London, Ontario, Canada, who met the following criteria: (1) a minimum of two years' experience in practice following qualification, and (2) having graduated since 1969. The size of this sample was 62. The two-year period was chosen because the transition from the more formal and structured environment of medical training to private practice is often accompanied by anxiety and uncertainty (Borus, 1982), and the restriction on year of graduation was to limit the age range of subjects and thereby partially eliminate the variability in their positions in the life cycle.

The mailing requested recipients to complete and return a questionnaire booklet consisting of six separate measures. To ensure a high return rate, the Dillman Total Design Method was utilized (Dillman, 1978). These measures consisted of the Cognition Check List, which measures anxiety and depression; the Coopersmith Self-Esteem Inventory, a measure of self-esteem; the People in Your Life Scale, designed to measure the quantity and quality of social supports; the Subjective Response to Stressful Life Events measure, which looks at the number of stressful events and the emotional response to them; the Work Response Questionnaire adapted from Yogev and Harris (1983), which measures work stress and work satisfaction; and finally, demographic data (Beck, Brown, Steer, Eidelson, & Riskind, 1987; Coopersmith, 1967; Marziali, 1987; Marziali & Pilkonis, 1986; Yogev & Harris, 1983). The purpose of these quantitative measures was to discriminate between those respondents who exhibited the highest incidence of psychological problems and those with the lowest.

Results

Fifty-two of the mailed questionnaires were returned, a response rate of 83.8%. Statistical analysis of the measures identified two variables as discriminating between symptomatic and nonsymptomatic respondents: self-esteem and intimate satisfaction (satisfaction with relationship with significant others). These two variables were correlated; in psychological terms, the quality of respondents' object relationships was reflected in their self-esteem. On the basis of these findings, those five respondents with the highest and those five with the lowest exhibition of self-esteem and positive object relationships were asked to participate in the next phase of the study.

PHASE II

Methodology

Phase II consisted of conducting semistructured interviews, developed by the author, with the 10 subjects identified above. The Separation Anxiety Test (SAT), designed by Hansburg (1980), was also administered. The purpose of the interview was to gather personal experiences of the subjects and elicit responses that revealed the nature of their perceptions of self and others. Subjects' responses were then rated on the dimensions of expansiveness, dependency, and detachment: These dimensions, taken from the work of Horney and Symonds, were selected to represent levels of resolution of separation-individuation, a precursor to identity formation, and are manifested in descriptions of the self in relation to others (Horney, 1945, 1950; Symonds, 1976, 1978, 1983). Expansiveness is defined as showing an orientation toward mastery, autonomy, and achievement; dependency, as showing a need for love and approval and appearing self-sacrificing and compliant. Detachment is defined as striving for self-sufficiency and the capacity to be alone.

The content areas of the interview included educational and occupational history, which was divided into three phases: premedicine, medical training, and medical practice. The next segment concerned itself with personal relationships, including family of origin and significant relationships. Again, the dimensions of dependency, detachment, and expansiveness were used to code each respondent's perceptions of herself and others. Sample questions dealing with educational-occupational history were: "Describe the kind of student you were during high school." Regarding family of origin, "Describe your relationship with your mother" . . . "How would she have described you?"

An attempt was made to examine the respondent's capacity to balance the personality dimensions of dependency, expansiveness, and detachment in areas that reflected her personal and professional life. For each respondent, three profiles were determined: a professional self-profile; a personal self-profile; and a profile combining both of these.

The Separation Anxiety Test (SAT) was also administered. This is a projective test, which assesses the emotional response to separation and loss, based on the principle that people's responses reflect the nature and quality of their object relations as they evolve through the process of separation-individuation. Its aim is to capture the balance between the achievement of individuality and the maintenance of attachment or connectedness to others.

The SAT consists of 12 black-and-white ink drawings that depict a child experiencing an event in which a separation occurs. Each picture is assigned a title, such as "The judge is placing the child in an institution," but the images are ambiguous enough to allow for the respondent's own interpretation of how the child might *feel*. The pictures are equally divided into two categories, mild and strong: Mild pictures depict a separation event that generates minimal separation stimulation, while the strong ones evoke a more intense emotional response. Accompanying each picture is a list of 17 statements that describe how the child is feeling or reacting to the separation experience, and the respondents select the ones that they think apply. In addition, they are asked whether such an event has ever happened to them, and if it has not, to imagine how it would feel if it had. The SAT provides both quantitative and qualitative scores; the qualitative focuses on the dimensions of individuation versus attachment, while the quantitative scores emphasize the degree or intensity of the emotional response to separation and loss.

Results

In the primary analysis of the data from Phase II, the information collected from each interview was compared to the results of the SAT, based on the dimensions of dependency, detachment, and expansiveness, and attachment versus individuation. These qualitative measures attempted to specifically identify some of the developmental antecedents that impact on the well-being of this group, particularly the process of separation-individuation.

Secondary analysis of the data will examine the relationship between the scores generated in Phase I, and the interview and SAT analysis from Phase II.

Conclusion

While the quantitative measures of Phase I were a necessary stepping-stone to Phase II, it is hoped that the qualitative findings of the latter may inform and enrich the earlier results. Ultimately, the two should enhance our understanding of the impact of developmental antecedents on the personal and professional well-being of this population.

References

Beck, A. T., Brown, G., Steer, R. A., Eidelson, J. I., & Riskind, J. H. (1987). Differentiating anxiety and depression: A test of the cognitive content-specificity hypothesis. *Journal of Abnormal Psychology, 96*(3), 197-183.

Blake, R. L., Jr. (1988). The Life-Space drawing as a measure of social relationships. *Family Medicine, 20*(4), 295-297.

Blake, R. L., Jr., & Vandiver, T. A. (1986). The reliability and validity of a ten-item measure of functional status. *Journal of Family Practice, 23*(5), 455-459.

Blishen, B. R., & McRoberts, H. A. (1971). A revised socioeconomic index for occupations in Canada. *Canadian Review of Social Anthropology, 34,* 50-59.

Borus, J. F. (1982). The transition to practice. *Journal of Medical Education, 57,* 593-601.

Chenitz, W. C., & Swanson, J. M. (1986). *From practice to grounded theory: Qualitative research in nursing.* Reading, MA: Addison-Wesley.

Coopersmith, S. (1967). *The antecedents of self-esteem.* San Francisco: Freeman.

Dillman, D. A. (1978). *Mail and telephone survey: The total design method.* New York: John Wiley.

Folstein, M. F., Folstein, S. E., & McHugh, P. R. (1975). Mini-mental state: A practical method for grading the cognitive mental state of patients for the clinician. *Journal of Psychiatric Research, 12,* 189-198.

Ford, A. B., Folmar, S. J., Salmon, R. B., Medalie, J. H., Roy, A. W., & Galazka, S. S. (1988). Health and function in the old and very old. *Journal of the American Geriatric Society, 36,* 187-197.

Glaser, B. G., & Strauss, A. L. (1967). *The discovery of grounded theory: Strategies for qualitative research*. Hawthorne, NY: Aldine.

Goldberg, D. P. (1972). *The detection of psychiatric illness by questionnaire*. London: Oxford University Press.

Goldberg, D. P., & Blackwell, B. (1970). Psychiatric illness in general practice: A detailed study using a new method of case identification. *British Medical Journal, 2*, 439-443.

Goldberg, D. P., & Hillier, V. F. (1979). A scaled version of the General Health Questionnaire. *Psychological Medicine, 9*, 139-145.

Gorden, R. L. (1980). *Interviewing: Strategy, techniques and tactics*. Homewood, IL: Dorsey.

Hansburg, H. G. (1980). *Separation disorders*. Huntington, NJ: Robert E. Krieger.

Holmes, T. H., & Rahe, R. H. (1967). The social readjustment rating scale. *Journal of Psychosomatic Research, 11*, 213-218.

Horney, K. (1945). *Our inner conflicts*. New York: W. W. Norton.

Horney, K. (1950). *Neurosis and human growth*. New York: W. W. Norton.

Horowitz, M., Wilner, N., & Alvarez, W. (1979). Impact of event scale: A measure of subjective stress. *Psychosomatic Medicine, 41*, 209-218.

Kaltreider, N. B., Wallace, A., & Horowitz, M. J. (1979). A field study of the stress response syndrome in young women after hysterectomy. *Journal of the American Medical Association, 242*, 1499-1503.

Kleinbaum, D. G., Kupper, L. L., & Morgenstern, H. (1982). *Epidemiological research: Principles and quantitative methods*. New York: Van Nostrand Reinhold.

Kruse, J. A., Thill-Baharozian, M. C., & Carlson, R. W. (1988). Comparison of clinical assessment with APACHE II for predicting mortality risk in patients admitted to a medical intensive care unit. *Journal of the American Medical Association, 260*, 1739-1742.

Kuzel, A. J. (1986). Naturalistic inquiry: An appropriate model for family medicine. *Family Medicine, 18*, 369-374.

Like, R. C., & Steiner, R. P. (1986). Medical anthropology and the family physician. *Family Medicine, 18*, 87-92.

Marziali, E. A. (1987). People in your life: Development of a social support measure for predicting psychotherapy outcome. *The Journal of Mental and Nervous Disease, 175*(6), 327-338.

Marziali, E. A., & Pilkonis, P. A. (1986, Spring). The measurement of subjective response to stressful life events. *Journal of Human Stress*, 5-12.

McGoldrick, M., & Gerson, R. (1986). *Genogram in family assessment*. New York: W. W. Norton.

Melzack, R., & Torgerson, W. B. (1971). On the language of pain. *Anesthesiology, 34*, 50-59.

Miles, M. B., & Huberman, A. M. (1984). *Qualitative data analysis: A sourcebook of new methods*. Newbury Park, CA: Sage.

Nuttal, S. (1988). *Pregnancy outcomes amoung a teenage sample*. Unpublished doctoral dissertation, The University of Western Ontario, London, Ontario.

Olson, D. H. (1986). Circumplex model VII: Validation studies and FACES III. *Family Process, 25*, 337-351.

O'Reilly, P. (1988). Methodological issues in social support and social network research. *Social Science and Medicine, 26*(8), 863-873.

Orth-Gomer, K., & Unden, A. (1987). The measurement of social support in population surveys. *Social Sciences and Medicine, 24*(1), 83-94.

Prince-Embury, S. (1984). The family health tree: A form for identifying physical symptom patterns within the family. *Journal of Family Practice, 18,* 75-81.

Reeb, K. G., Graham, A. V., Zyzanski, S. J., & Kitson, G. C. (1987). Predicting low birthweight and complicated labor in urban black women: A biopsychosocial perspective. *Social Sciences and Medicine, 25*(12), 1321-1327.

Schatzman, L., & Strauss, A. L. (1973). *Field research: Strategies for a natural sociology.* Englewood Cliffs, NJ: Prentice-Hall.

Scrimshaw, S. C., & Hurtado, E. (1988). Anthropological involvement in the Central American diarrheal disease control project. *Social Sciences and Medicine, 27,* 97-105.

Seeman, T. E., & Berkman, L. F. (1988). Structural characteristics of social networks and relationship with social support in the elderly: Who provides support. *Social Sciences and Medicine, 26*(7), 737-749.

Stange, K. C., & Zyzanski, S. J. (1989). Integrating qualitative and quantitative research methods. *Family Medicine, 21,* 448-451.

Stiles, W. B. (1978). Verbal response models and dimensions of interpersonal roles: A method of discourse analysis. *Journal of Personality and Social Psychology, 36,* 693-703.

Stiles, W. B., Putnam, S. M., James, S. A., & Wolf, M. H. (1979). Dimensions of patient and physician roles in medical screening Interviews. *Social Science and Medicine, 13,* 335-341.

Strauss, A. L. (1987). *Qualitative analysis for social scientists.* New York: Cambridge University Press.

Swanson-Kauffman, K. (1983). *The unborn one: A profile of the human experience of miscarriage.* Unpublished doctoral thesis, The University of Colorado, Denver.

Symonds, A. (1976). Neurotic dependency in successful women. *Journal of American Academy of Psychoanalysis, 4*(1), 95-103.

Symonds, A. (1978). The psychodynamics of expansiveness in success-oriented women. *American Journal of Psychoanalysis, 38,* 195-206.

Symonds, A. (1983). Emotional conflicts of the career women: Women in medicine. *American Journal of Psychoanalysis, 43*(1), 21-37.

Tennen, H., & Herzberger, S. (1985). Impact of event scale. In D. J. Keyser & R. C. Sweetland (Eds.), *Test critiques.* Kansas City, MO: Test Corporation of America.

Turner, R. J. (1983). Direct, indirect and moderating effects of social support upon psychological distress and associated conditions. In H. B. Kaplan (Ed.), *Psychosocial stress.* New York: Academic Press.

Turner, R. J., Frankel, B. G., & Levin, D. (1983). Social support: Conceptualization measurement and implications for mental health. In J. R. Greenley (Ed.), *Research in community and mental health* (Vol. III). Greenwich, CT: JAI Press.

Wolf, M. H., Putnam, S. M., James, S. A., & Stiles, W. B. (1978). The medical interview satisfaction scale: Development of a scale to measure patient perception of physician behavior. *Journal of Behavioral Medicine, 1,* 390-401.

Yogev, S., & Harris, S. (1983). Women physicians during residency years: Work-load, work satisfaction and self concept. *Social Science and Medicine, 17*(12), 837-841.

Zilberg, N. J., Weiss, D. S., & Horowitz, M. J. (1982). Impact of event scale: A cross-validation study and some empirical evidence supporting a conceptual model of stress response syndromes. *Journal of Consulting and Clinical Psychology, 50,* 407-414.

12 Primary Care Nursing: A Model for Research

TOULA M. GERACE

Introduction

Nurses who work in primary health care settings, while they may have diverse educational and experiential backgrounds, share common philosophies in caring for individuals and families from infancy to old age. They are alternately referred to as primary care nurses, family practice nurses, or nurse practitioners (Registered Nurses' Association of Ontario, 1980). As generalists who work in association with other members of multidisciplinary health care teams (Brunetto & Birk, 1972), they have developed expertise in such areas as maternal-child health, growth and development, health education and counseling, and family-focused care.

The hallmarks of primary care nursing are the restoration, maintenance, and promotion of health through all stages of the life span. Health promotion or primary prevention is the most characteristic feature, although secondary and tertiary prevention are becoming equally important. Since the chance of encountering ill health increases with age, the burgeoning elderly population will potentially expose primary health care providers to greater numbers of unhealthy people requiring secondary and tertiary preventive strategies. By caring for individuals and families over the continuum of time, the primary nurse is in an ideal position to understand the patients' experiences of disease as well as of health, and to make appropriate interventions. Such interventions include knowledge of and recommendations for currently accepted screening procedures, anticipatory guidance regarding diagnostic interventions, interpretation of therapeutic decisions, advocacy at all levels of care, monitoring recovery and rehabilitation from disease, and assisting patients to achieve and cope with altered levels of functioning.

In understanding the whole person, in the context of family, society, culture and environment, primary care nurses can apply broader definitions to health and illness. The narrow view that health is simply the absence of disease, thereby inferring that health promotion only means preventing disease, is not compatible with such an understanding. Health is a state of mind, as well as body, and incorporates environmental, cultural, and family belief systems. A definition of health must embody what a person is as well as what he or she might become. It must be based on realistic possibilities for the individual to potentially live the experience of health as a state of well-being (Benner & Wrubel, 1989). Based on such a definition, health promotion, or the development of healthy living, becomes personalized rather than generalized. Illness has similarly contextual meaning; it is the unique, personal experience of perceived abnormality, and cannot be equated to disease. Consequently, the notion of disease prevention is also too narrow in scope: Illness prevention is much more appropriate.

The nursing process, a basic problem-solving process that includes stages of assessment, planning, implementation, and evaluation, is incorporated into functions carried out by nurses working in primary health care settings. Broad role categories of primary care nurses are as follows:

- *Coordinator:* This includes making suitable referrals to appropriate health care providers and resources after assessing the nature of the patient's concern. Coordination of care occurs at multiple levels: the individual, the family, the immediate primary care system, and the general health care system.
- *Educator:* This includes determining the health education needs of patients and acting as a facilitator in providing health education strategies and resources. Anticipatory guidance is also considered to be a type of health education.
- *Communicator:* This includes communicating with patients in person or by telephone. Patient concerns are then communicated and

interpreted to physicians and other pertinent health care providers, as determined by the nature of the concern. Counseling is another form of communication.

- *Patient Advocate:* This includes speaking to systems, whether they be family, social, or health care, on behalf of the patient.

The role of the nurse in primary care is a diverse and often ambiguous one. It sometimes seems as though very little is being done unless something can be measured objectively and physically, such as changing dressings, doing physical assessments, or giving injections. However, coordinating care, teaching, and speaking to and on behalf of patients are often the most important functions of primary care nurses. They represent the avenues toward fully understanding the whole person and his or her health concerns, as well as providing guidance for nursing care.

The Primary Care Team

Primary care nurses work principally with primary care physicians. Their role has been described by Allen (1983) as the more traditional one of *assistant,* which involves carrying out tasks delegated by the physician, and *replacement* of the physician, which involves carrying out some or most of the same tasks as the physician to fill gaps in the health care system. The latter has been described by Murphy (1970) as role extension.

A third and perhaps more suitable model is a collaborative one in which nurses function independently, dependently, and, most important, interdependently with physicians (Aradine & Pridham, 1973). Murphy (1970) describes this as role expansion. Alt-White, Charns, and Strayer (1983) have defined nurse-physician collaboration as the process whereby nurses and physicians work together in the delivery of care, jointly contributing in a balanced relationship characterized by mutual trust. Essential to this model is a nonhierarchical system of communication and responsibility. Viewed generically as the common environment in which physicians and nurses have independent as well as overlapping functions, the primary care setting will provide ownership to both professions, resulting in a mutual commitment to a specific shared practice population. Thus, primary care nurses and physicians can function in a complementary fashion. As coproviders of care, they offer a comprehensive "package" of health care that incorporates expertise from both nursing and medicine. Elpern, Rodts, DeWald, and West (1983) have defined this working relationship as *associated practice*, stressing that it is a practice arrangement that is voluntary, negotiated, and collegial.

The ideal practice setting is one in which there is a multidisciplinary health care team, consisting of a primary care physician and nurse forming the core of the team, and members of other health disciplines working in close association. As Given and Simmons (1977) describe it, patient care is approached by team members on the basis of joint problem formulation, data collection, and goal setting in determining team activities to achieve problem solution.

Collaboration among professionals is necessary if a team is to function effectively. Devereux (1981) cites three essential components for collaborative practice: communication, competence, and accountability. Open and honest communication is imperative in promoting productive, contributory dialogue between and among professionals in order to maximize patient care; in addition, all members of the team must be aware of what the others' thoughts and/or actions are regarding identified problems, whether they be related to patients, each other, or team functioning. Clinical competence is important in establishing the requisite mutual trust of collaborative practice; team members must be able to rely on and have confidence in one another's clinical knowledge and skills. Accountability entails responsibility for actions taken regarding patient-care decisions; members of the team are accountable on a personal level as well as to each other regarding decisions made independently or collectively. Other important components of collaboration include assertiveness, respect for other professionals' contributions, and the ability to negotiate (Puta, 1989).

Theoretical Considerations

The purpose of any clinical theory is to generate and expand knowledge and guide professional behavior by using sound principles stemming from a theoretical base. The foundation of current nursing theory was established by Florence Nightingale (1859/1946) when she outlined the principles of disease prevention, recovery from illness, and the importance of the patient's environment. She envisaged nursing as a profession with a distinct knowledge base. But it was not until the 1950s and 1960s that nurses began to develop their own distinct theories. Educational programs were expanding and nurses were developing a greater sense of identity. They wanted to clearly define the nature of nursing, as well as promote and communicate its professional status to one another, the public, and other health care professionals (Whall, 1989). Up until this time nursing practice, although guided by principles developed by nurses, also relied heavily on borrowed theories from other disciplines, particularly those of medicine and the social sciences. Examples of borrowed theories especially useful in primary care are systems theory in evaluating families, well or ill, in social and environmental contexts; developmental theory in assessing behavior; needs theory in understanding human behavior related to health and illness; and educational theory in developing strategies for health education and intervention. Meleis (1985) has suggested that borrowed theories become shared theories as they go through a process of integration and synthesis when used within a nursing context. Although shared, the derivation of the theory is not from a nursing base. In this sense the discipline of nursing, as a separate and explicit one, is not advanced.

The purpose of developing a nursing theory is to describe the process of nursing care, and thereby prescribe effective strategies of care by providing nurses with goals for assessment, diagnosis, and intervention (Meleis, 1985). In addition, theory will direct research efforts in defining, refining, and exploring questions pertinent to establishing nursing as an independent discipline. Theories also need to be tested through research in order to establish their reliability and validity before they can be adopted for practice. As Kidd and Morrison (1988) have explained, the goal of practice, theory, and research is to integrate knowledge to arrive at ultimate meaning.

Four concepts central to all nursing theories are those of person, environment, health, and nursing. These are therefore components of those theories that are applicable to primary care nursing. Although there is no one theory geared solely to this area, there are two that lend themselves well to it: the Neuman Systems Model and the Allen Nursing Model.

The Neuman model (Lancaster & Whall, 1989) focuses on individual or group response to stressors, and upon nursing intervention in assisting the system to respond to stressors. It is particularly useful to primary care nursing as it incorporates primary, secondary, and tertiary levels of prevention. It also provides a structure to analyze, understand, and evaluate the experience of both altered and normal levels of functioning.

The Allen Nursing Model (Kravitz & Frey, 1989) focuses on the contribution of nurses to health as primary providers of care, with particular emphasis on health promotion. Although illness is considered, the major emphasis is on health, which may prohibit the evaluation of illness in primary care. The family, within its social context, is the center of care. Evaluating the potential for learning and promoting healthy behavior is stressed. This model has been tested in primary health care settings, and is shaping the thinking of health scientists. It is particularly useful when evaluating the structure and function of primary care nursing.

Nursing theories are continuing to develop and evolve; therefore, all nursing research may not yet be linked to current theory. It is imperative that the process of nursing be described in order to understand the practice; thereby guiding theory development and research.

Primary Care Nursing Research

Primary care is an excellent setting for nursing research and has a tremendous potential for this. The practice population, usually composed of a stable number of patients and their families, constitutes a wide range of health and health problems from infancy to old age. This stability, coupled with the longitudinal relationships established between patients and nurses, offers a unique opportunity to study areas of interest over time. The environment is particularly suitable to evaluate the outcome of health care interventions.

In addition, just as the primary care setting is opportune for collaborative practice, it is also ideal for collaborative research between nurses, physicians, and other health care providers. The composition of the research team is directly related to the type of research question posed; for example, it might include physicians, nurses, and social workers in studying the dynamics and functioning of single parent families. Principles of collaborative research are as follows:

- *Collaborative Practice:* Collaborative practice-based research offers an opportunity to ask and answer questions related to a specific shared population. Varying levels of experience with research, as well as acknowledged professional differences, allow for an eclectic approach to the research process. This also gives the more experienced researcher an opportunity to act as a mentor to those with less experience, thereby enhancing the growth and development of the research team.
- *Commitment:* Physical and emotional commitment to the research project are essential if it is to be carried through to completion. Being committed to the research team can enhance motivation, which at times lags. Differences in work styles, abilities, and goals need to be acknowledged at the outset in determining whether the team can approach an area of study.
- *Communication:* As in collaborative practice, communication needs to be open and honest regarding the question asked, the methodology used, and the interpretation of results. In addition, determining levels of authorship, a sensitive issue, must be decided upon before commencing any project.

Primary care nursing research is essential to describe, define, and develop the practice-theory-research link. Fawcett (1989) emphasized that descriptive studies that examine characteristics of an individual, group, situation, or event are required when nothing or very little is known about a particular occurrence. She also stresses that replicating studies is necessary to establish the generalizability of findings to various settings and groups of people. Because much of nursing practice, particularly in primary care, centers around meaningful interactions with patients, qualitative rather than quantitative research may be more appropriate in ultimately developing theories directly related to primary care nursing.

There are five broad areas of study to be considered in primary care nursing research: health, illness, family, education, and roles:

- *Health:* As previously described, the restoration, maintenance, and promotion of health is a basic tenet of primary care nursing. In order to provide effective care in this area, it is imperative that we gain a better understanding of personal meanings of health, as well as health-seeking behavior. In addition, evaluation studies of health promotion strategies are needed. Several examples of such studies are presented below.

Nutritional assessment and counseling is a common area of expertise for primary care nurses. But do we really know why patients desire to lose weight? White (1984), in a qualitative examination of a group of patients entering a weight loss program, found that body image was far more important than were health concerns to these patients in their decision to lose weight. A greater understanding of the obese individual was achieved, resulting in a much more definitive recommendation to assess this problem more completely—rather than advising patients to lose weight for health reasons only, as many health care providers often do.

It has been suggested that primary care nurses are amply qualified to carry out well baby care, but the reaction of mothers to this has often been overlooked. A study by Christie, Janzen, and Stewart (1983) found that mothers perceived the nurse to be as important as the doctor in well baby care, and preferred to speak to the nurse over the telephone regarding problems that arose.

Primary care nurses are also very much involved in the prenatal care of patients. Patterson, Freese, and Goldenberg (1990) conducted a grounded theory study to explore how women utilize health care during pregnancy. Most of the 27 women interviewed had sought prenatal care. Commonly held expectations were that prenatal care could provide information, reassurance, medications, and early detection and treatment of problems. The major concern of the women was seeking safe passage through pregnancy and childbirth. Processes used to achieve this were seeking out care, consulting, transferring, waiting, contingency planning, and self-care. In so understanding the experience of pregnancy, interventions that will meet the needs and expectations of patients can be employed.

Immunization is another area of primary care expertise. How can immunization rates be improved? In a study evaluating an outreach strategy (Gerace & Sangster, 1988), the currently held 20% immunization rate for influenza vaccine was increased to almost 70%. The outreach was found to be successful in achieving an improved rate of immunization, findings supported by other, similar studies (Larson, Olsen, Coles, & Shertell, 1979; McDowell, Newell, & Rosser, 1986). Analogous to this was a study of the rubella status of women from one practice population (Gerace, 1987). Those found to be susceptible were identified and actively immunized in an attempt to prevent the tragedy of the Congenital Rubella Syndrome.

- *Illness:* Patterns of illness need to be examined in order to gain an understanding of early morbidity, illness behavior, and individual and family coping mechanisms.

A primary care multiphased qualitative investigation of patient perspectives of health care relationships in chronic illness was carried out by Thorne and Robinson (1989). It confirmed that such relationships evolve over time through three predictable stages: naive trust, disenchantment, and guarded alliance. Such findings have the potential to facilitate a focused assessment from which health care providers can negotiate plans to create and account for satisfying relationships with their chronically ill patients.

Utz, Hammer, Whitmire, and Grass (1990) interviewed 20 patients with diagnosed Mitral Valve Prolapse (MVP) regarding self-care needs. The majority described experiences indicating that their perceptions of body image and health status were affected by the diagnosis of MVP. Although all the participants continued normal activities of daily living, 90% made comments that reflected altered body image, while all felt their health was altered as well. Although MVP is not considered to be a serious disease, the women in this study were experiencing the illness, supporting the contextual difference between disease and illness.

- *Family:* Knowledge of family systems with respect to health and illness concerns is an integral component of primary care nursing, yet this is an area lacking in research (Friedman, 1986). The role of the primary care nurse within the context of the family has not been examined, and only recently has an interest developed in this (Murphy, 1986; Robertson & Stewart, 1985). In order to develop theoretical models for primary care nursing of families, research is not only recommended but required.

• *Education:* Patient education is an area in which primary care nurses have gained proficiency. In order to optimize patient care, the describing, testing and evaluating of educational strategies and materials is essential. Additionally, in family medicine teaching programs nurses often provide both formal and informal education to residents. It is crucial that such involvement be described and evaluated to provide guidance to other nurses entering similar environments.

There have been few studies addressing patient education in primary care (Geyman, 1980). One such study (Miller & Shank, 1986) compared the effectiveness of three methods of presenting the same patient education: (1) a physician plus educational material, (2) a nurse plus educational material, and (3) the educational material alone. Post-intervention knowledge and compliance of patients were compared to that of patients who had received no educational intervention. It was found that having nurses present the educational material resulted in equal effectiveness in knowledge gained by patients as compared to physicians presenting it, but there was greater effectiveness in follow-up compliance. The use of educational materials alone did not result in increased knowledge and only slightly improved compliance. Such findings support the significant role that primary care nurses can have in patient education.

Dawson-Saunders and Wylie (1988) carried out a survey of nurses involved in medical education in the United States and Canada to determine how they were contributing to it. They found that departments of internal medicine, education, and community medicine were more likely to include nurses as teachers than were departments of psychiatry, surgery, and family practice. This result seems surprising because there is, at least, an impression that primary care nurses are very much involved in medical education. One of the limitations of this study, however, is that its information came from asking departmental chairpersons to name nurses involved in education—not from asking the nurses themselves. In order to get accurate representation and information it would be preferable that the nurses identify and describe their roles themselves.

- *Roles:* Primary care nurses have a multitude of roles. It is essential that these be researched so that nurses as well as other health care providers can understand them; so that the nursing role can be develop and further defined; and so that collegial relationships can have a grounded basis for interaction. There has been very little systematic study of team interaction reported in the literature (Feiger & Schmitt, 1979), and few studies examining nurse-physician relationships and their impact on patient care (Weiss & Davis, 1985). Primary care provides an ideal setting in which to explore both these areas.

For example, a major role of nurses in primary care is telephone care, but do we really understand telephone encounters? A group of nurses recorded their telephone contacts for two one-week periods (Gerace & Huffman, in press). It was found that the majority of calls took place on Mondays, in the afternoon, and were five minutes or less in length. Most of the encounters were regarding adult medical problems, and the three most prevalent management strategies dealt with medications, reassurance and support, and health teaching. While the nurses felt positive about most encounters, this feeling was strongest when using management strategies of health teaching, reassurance and support, and counseling to deal with problems of social-emotional concerns, maternal-child health, and communicable disease. They did not feel significantly positive about medical problems, which constituted 68% of the encounters. Another important finding was that only 35% of the calls were documented in patient charts.

If nursing research is to grow in primary care, specific questions pertaining to the role and function of nurses in this setting, in relation to current theoretical models of nursing, will ultimately have to be answered. Additionally, primary care nurses need to undertake studies that assess the quality of their care, based on components of nursing practice. To rely on other professions to do this for them raises concern that (1) a clear identity of primary care nursing will never develop; (2) nurses will be misrepresented because of misunderstood role differentiation and outcome evaluations based on other professions' standards, behaviors, and expectations; (3) a hierarchical system of research will develop, paralleling other hierarchical systems of primary care; and (4) the research needs of the nursing profession will not be met. It is imperative that nurses be encouraged to partake in the research process at whatever level is possible—whether it be in developing critical inquiry in asking researchable questions, partaking in projects, or independently or collaboratively carrying out investigations.

References

Allen, M. (1983). Primary care nursing: Research in action. In L. Hockey (Ed.), *Recent advances in nursing: Primary care nursing*. Edinburgh: Churchill Livingstone.

Alt-White, A. C., Charns, M., & Strayer, R. (1983). Personal, organizational and managerial factors related to nurse-physician collaboration. *Nursing Administration Quarterly, 8*, 8-18.

Aradine, C. R., & Pridham, K. F. (1973). Model for collaboration. *Nursing Outlook, 21*, 655-657.

Benner, P., & Wrubel, J. (1989). *The primacy of caring: Stress and coping in health and illness*. New York: Addison-Wesley.

Brunetto, R., & Birk, P. (1972). The primary care nurse: The generalist in a structured health team. *American Journal of Public Health, 62*, 6-8.

Christie, R., Janzen, I., & Stewart, M. (1983). Well baby care: The nurse's job. *Canadian Family Physician, 29*, 927-932.

Dawson-Saunders, B., & Wylie, N. (1988). A survey of nurses in medical education. In *The role of the nurse in clinical medical education*. Southern Illinois University School of Medicine.

Devereux, P. M. (1981). Does joint practice work? *The Journal of Nursing Administration, 11*(6), 39-43.

Elpern, E. H., Rodts, M. F., DeWald, R. L., & West, J. W. (1983). Associated practice: A case for professional collaboration. *The Journal of Nursing Administration, 13*(11), 27-31.

Fawcett, J. (1989, June). A declaration of nursing independence: The relation of theory and research to nursing practice. *The Journal of Nursing Administration,* 36-39.

Feiger, S. M., & Schmitt, M. H. (1979). Collegiality in interdisciplinary health teams: Its measurement and its effects. *Social Science and Medicine, 13*, 217-229.

Friedman, M. M. (1986). *Family nursing: Theory and assessment* (2nd ed.). Norwalk, CT: Appleton-Century-Crofts.

Gerace, T. M. (1987). Rubella screening and immunization: An ongoing challenge. *Canadian Family Physician, 33*, 111-115.

Gerace, T. M., & Huffman, M. C. (in press). Family practice nurses and the telephone. *Canadian Family Physician*.

Gerace, T. M., & Sangster, J. F. (1988). Influenza vaccination: A comparison of two outreach strategies. *Family Medicine, 20*(11), 43-45.

Geyman, J. P. (1980). How effective is patient education? *Journal of Family Practice, 10*, 973-974.

Given, B., & Simmons, S. (1977). The interdisciplinary health-care team: Fact or fiction? *Nursing Forum, 16*(2), 165-184.

Kidd, P., & Morrison, E. F. (1988). The progression of knowledge in nursing: A search for meaning. *Image: Journal of Nursing Scholarship, 20*(4), 222-224.

Kravitz, M., & Frey, M. A. (1989). The Allen nursing model. In J. Fitzpatrick & A. Whall (Eds.), *Conceptual models of nursing: Analysis an application* (2nd ed.). Norwalk, CT: Appleton & Lange.

Lancaster, D. R., & Whall, A. L. (1989). The Neuman systems model. In J. Fitzpatrick & A. Whall (Eds.), *Conceptual models of nursing: Analysis and application*. Norwalk, CT: Appleton & Lange.

Larson, E. B., Olsen, E., Cole, W., & Shertell, S. (1979). The relationship of health beliefs and a postcard reminder to influenza vaccination. *Journal of Family Practice, 8*, 1207-1211.

McDowell, I., Newell, C., & Rosser, W. (1986). Comparison of three methods of recalling patients for influenza vaccination. *Canadian Medical Association Journal, 135*, 991-997.

Meleis, A. I. (1985). *Theoretical nursing: Development & progress*. Philadelphia: J. B. Lippincott.

Miller, G., & Shank, C. (1986). Patient education: Comparative effectiveness by means of presentation. *Journal of Family Practice, 22*(2), 178-181.

Murphy, J. F. (1970). Role expansion or role extension: Some conceptual differences. *Nursing Forum, 9*(4), 380-390.

Murphy, S. (1986). Family study and nursing research. *Image: Journal of Nursing Scholarship, 18*(4), 171-174.

Nightingale, F. (1946). *Notes on nursing: What it is and what it is not*. Philadelphia: J. B. Lippincott (Facsimile of the First Edition, printed in London, 1859).

Patterson, E. T., Freese, M. P., & Goldenberg, R. L. (1990). Seeking safe passage: Utilizing health care during pregnancy. *Image: Journal of Nursing Scholarship, 22*(1), 27-31.

Puta, D. F. (1989). Nurse-physician collaboration toward quality. *Journal of Nursing Quality Assurance, 3*(2), 11-18.

Registered Nurses' Association of Ontario. (1980). *Statement on the role and function of the primary care nurse*. Toronto: RNAO.

Robertson, D. L., & Stewart, T. J. (1985). Families and health: A review of clinical and research issues for primary care. *Family Practice Research Journal, 4*(3), 42-50.

Thorne, S. E., & Robinson, C. A. (1989). Guarded alliance: Health care relationships in chronic illness. *Image: Journal of Nursing Scholarship, 21*(3), 153-157.

Utz, S. W., Hammer, J., Whitmire, V. M., & Grass, S. (1990). Perceptions of body image and health status in persons with mitral valve prolapse. *Image: Journal of Nursing Scholarship, 22*(1), 19-22.

Weiss, S. J., & Davis, H. P. (1985). Validity and reliability of the collaborative practice scales. *Nursing Research, 34*, 299-305.

Whall, A. L. (1989). Nursing theory issues and debates. In J. Fitzpatrick & A. Whall (Eds.), *Conceptual models of nursing: Analysis and application* (2nd ed.). Norwalk, CT: Appleton & Lange.

White, J. (1984). The relationship of clinical practice and research. *Journal of Advanced Nursing, 9,* 181-187.

13 Primary Health Care— A Nursing Model: A Danish-Newfoundland (Canada) Project

DOROTHY C. HALL
ABRAHAM S. ROSS
DANA EDGE
GARFIELD A. PYNN

Background to the Project

Many countries are currently searching for innovative ways to reduce the cost of health services without lowering their quality or availability. Canada and Denmark are no exception: Both countries are engaged in seeking sound methods of maintaining and improving health services, without engendering an insupportable increase in costs.

It is well accepted internationally that one of the best ways to achieve this goal is to help individuals, families, and communities attain and retain optimal physical, psychological, and social health, as opposed to providing care only after they become ill or injured. One of the most credible methods of doing this is to reshape our current sickness-oriented health services into a three-tier system made up of primary, secondary, and tertiary subsystems (see Figure 13.1).

The World Health Organization (WHO), of which Canada and Denmark are founding members, has for more than 20 years been urging its member countries to adopt and develop such a system, often referred to as a health services pyramid. Chronic and acute

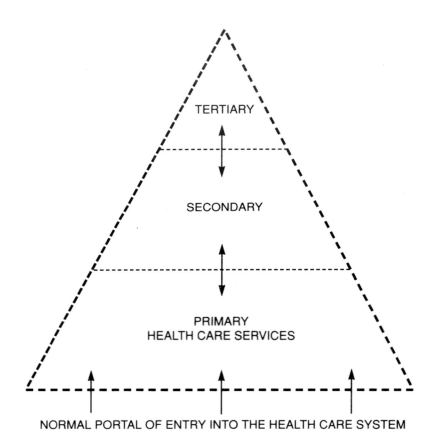

Table 13.1. Comprehensive Health Services System

health care services of increasing technological complexity are found at the second and third levels of the pyramid, while the primary health care subsystem forms the base. WHO documents state that good primary care is "an integral part both of the Country's health system . . . and of the overall social and economic development of the Community"; that it is "based on practical, scientifically sound . . . methods and technology"; that it is acceptable, accessible, and accountable to the people it serves; and that it "is provided at a cost that the community can afford to maintain at every stage of (its) development" (WHO, 1984). Primary health care provides *promotive, preventive, curative, supportive,* and *rehabilitative* health services, with emphasis placed on keeping individuals and communities well, on promoting and supporting good self-care and family care, and on developing self-reliance and self-determination regarding health (see Fig. 13.2).

Canada and Denmark were among the many countries that participated in the 1978 WHO/UNICEF-sponsored international conference on primary health care in Alma Ata, USSR, and collaborated in the preparation of what became known as the Alma Ata Declaration. At this conference, it was agreed that primary health care should be "the main thrust and focus for the promotion of world health" (WHO, 1984).

To date however, most of the countries that supported the concepts put forward at the Alma Ata Conference have found it difficult, for a variety of reasons, to introduce primary health care services that meet the criteria described above. One major problem has revolved around identifying the health care worker who could best implement all the components of good primary health care at an affordable cost. In 1985 Dr. Halfdan Mahler, then Director General of WHO, suggested that the worker who comes closest to meeting these requirements is the nurse. In many countries nurses are already prepared both by education and experience to provide services that range from prevention and promotion, through simple curative care, and into the areas of rehabilitative and supportive services. There is, therefore, little doubt that if nurses are provided with requisite support—attitudinal, legal, educational, and resource-based—they could provide the kind of primary health care that so many countries need.

Canadian and Danish nurses have already demonstrated their ability to give this kind of multifaceted care: in Canada, through the outpost services that are the backbone of health care in the North, and in Denmark, through comprehensive home care programs. These programs, operated, in many instances around the clock, are an integral and important component of the Danish primary health care services subsystem, as are the longstanding

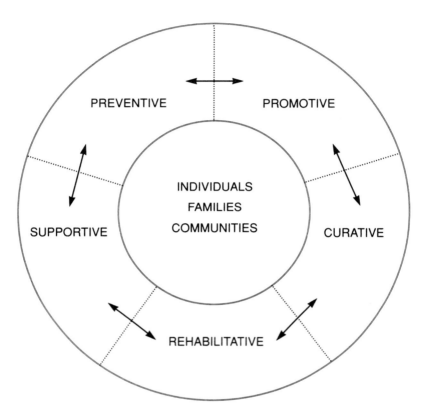

Table 13.2. Primary Health Care—Comprehensive Health Services

public health nursing services to families. The impact of the latter has been demonstrated through a pronounced decline in the infant mortality rate over the past 50 years.

However, a primary health care service that provides all facets of comprehensive health services to all age groups, as described by WHO, does not yet exist in either Denmark or Canada. In addition, there is a dearth of good nursing research in the primary care setting. What is needed is not only a demonstration of primary health care services by nurses, but also well-designed research that can evaluate these services in terms of implementation, process, impact on the health status of the population served, and cost-effectiveness.

The Danish-Canadian Primary Health Care Project

INTRODUCTION

The Primary Health Care Project was conceived and developed by a group of Danish and Canadian nurses, who came together in 1985 to discuss the role of nurses in providing primary health care services in the community. This group, finding the model put forward at Alma Ata challenging and worth exploring further, approached their respective professional associations: the Association of Registered Nurses of Newfoundland (ARNN) and the Danish Nurses Organization (DNO). Both associations agreed that a bilateral, primary health care project should be jointly developed, and set aside funds for this purpose.

Work began in earnest with the appointment of two project directors, one at the offices of the Association of Registered Nurses of Newfoundland and the other at the Danish Institute for Health and Nursing Research in Copenhagen. One of the founding members of the project, a retired WHO Regional Officer for Nursing who was familiar with both Danish and Canadian health services, was appointed the international project coordinator.

PURPOSE

The Project can most accurately be described as a "demonstration project," whose overall purpose is to effect a measurable improvement in the health of selected communities in Denmark and Newfoundland through the provision of primary health care services managed and largely provided by nurses. It will aim at:

- effecting a measurable improvement in the health status of individuals and families served by the Project;
- effecting a measurable improvement in health directed lifestyles;
- identifying environmental health hazards and working with the community to reduce or eliminate them;

- demonstrating a cost-effective way of using resources to provide promotive, preventive, curative, rehabilitative, and supportive services to meet the basic health needs;
- giving special attention to the health care needs of high-risk groups such as the elderly, the disabled, mothers and children, the chronically ill, and persons in high-risk occupations;
- demonstrating that nurses can provide safe and effective primary health care services in an affordable and cost-effective manner;
- involving the community in program planning, implementation, and evaluation;
- providing around-the-clock services, 365 days a year, in the home, school, workplace, or clinic;
- developing a prototype of primary health care services that could be usefully modeled not only in other regional communities but around the world;
- conducting relevant research studies on ways to improve care;
- collaborating with other health care providers to ensure that the most appropriate care is provided to clients and that good working relationships are operative;
- assisting individuals and groups to acquire knowledge and to develop skills in personal, family, and community health care.

The foregoing will be achieved by providing the selected communities with the kind of primary health care services envisioned in the Alma Ata Declaration. As stated, these services will be managed and largely provided by nurses. However, their administration, planning, implementation, and evaluation will be carried out in close collaboration and cooperation with members of the community served and with local workers in other health disciplines.

It is expected that every community in which the Project is implemented will elect or appoint some type of community council or board to act in an advisory capacity. Linkages will be established with relevant persons and/or institutions at the secondary and tertiary levels of the health care system, but encouragement of self-determination and self-care with regard to health will be a cornerstone.

The principles and concepts that guide all phases and levels of Project development are the following:

1. the WHO concepts of primary health care as expressed in the Alma Ata Declaration and further developed in numerous WHO publications;

2. the concepts of nursing as put forward in the 1979 *A Position Paper on Nursing* by D.C. Hall, the 1988 Report of the WHO/EURO European Conference on Nursing and WHA 30.48, WHA 36.1, WHA 42.27;

3. the development of a *partnership of equals* among workers from all disciplines providing health services and between these workers and the public they serve.

In addition to implementation, the design provides for overall evaluation of the Project and the individual practices (described below). It also offers opportunities for service-based studies and research, maintains in-service education for practice staff, and provides health education for the public. The educational component should be of interest to schools of nursing and medicine and to any individuals or groups concerned with the development of primary health care services.

The Project and the Practice

Development of the Project will involve two closely related yet discrete sets of activities: one set conducted at Project level, and the other at the individual Practice level. These activities, which include both one-time and ongoing tasks, are illustrated in Figure 13.3.

Practices will employ the "primary nursing" method, a well-defined system whereby all individuals or families requiring care have their own nurse, just as they would a personal or family physician. This individual is called the *primary nurse*, and the total number of clients for whom she (or he) provides care is referred to as the *caseload*. Primary nurses are accountable to both their clients and their peers for the outcomes of this care, which invests them with the authority and related responsibility to assess health needs, plan the care to be provided, ensure that the plan is implemented, and evaluate the outcomes of the interventions. This sequence of actions is known as the *nursing process.*

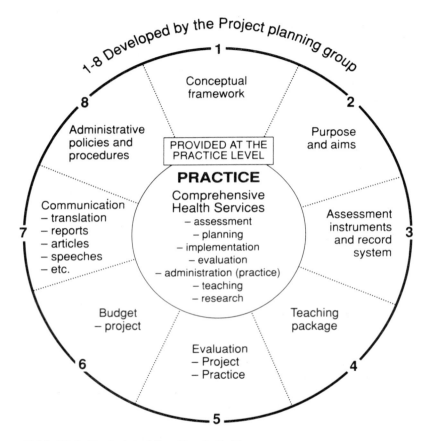

Table 13.3. Project and Practice Activities

Each Practice will be initiated in its community under the leadership of a nurse who is designated local Project Coordinator. This individual, along with other nurses in the Practice, will be expected to carry a caseload. Nurses will use Project-prescribed instruments and methods to assess, plan for, evaluate, and document care. Current ethical and nursing care standards applicable to Denmark and Newfoundland will apply respectively in each national Practice.

State-of-the-art quality control, maintenance, and assurance methods will be as described in Project documents and will be taught in the in-service staff education. These will include the use of concurrent and retroactive record audits and the assessment of outcomes in terms of the individuals or groups served, caregivers, and of the overall system of which the Practice is a part. "Outcomes" are health-directed goals that are mutually developed and agreed upon between the primary nurse and the client, and may relate to physical, mental, or social parameters. Goals may be approached through the development and achievement of a series of subgoals that are time-targeted and achievable with the resources available. Audits will be done to ensure that appropriate goals and subgoals are set and achieved within the determined time frame.

In addition, nurses in the Practice will be encouraged to initiate and carry out service-based research studies.

IMPLEMENTATION

Once an agreement has been reached between a community, the International Steering Committee, and the appropriate national bodies, the steps in implementing a Practice are as follows:

- collection of baseline data by the Project evaluation team;
- selection and appointment of the local Project Coordinator and the Practice nursing staff. Where applicable, planning for integration into the project model of traditional community nursing services should also begin at this step.
- planned and active involvement of the community and its citizens in the Practice; establishment of an advisory Primary Health Care Practice Council or Board;
- selection and appointment of support staff: secretarial, housekeeping, and so forth;
- setting up the Primary Health Care Centre;
- in-service education of nursing and related personnel in the Practice. During this period the health needs of the community will be assessed and decisions will be made regarding which needs should be addressed.

- formal opening of the Primary Health Care Centre and start of active services. All three levels of service (individual, family, and community) should be available from the onset, as should the availability of all required promotive, preventive, curative, rehabilitative, and supportive services.

Linkages with other health workers and with the secondary and tertiary levels of the health care system should be in place before the Practice starts.

Evaluation

Evaluation will be conducted at both the Project and Practice levels. The former will be carried out by "at arm's length" teams of evaluators in both the Canadian and Danish settings.

EVALUATION AT THE PROJECT LEVEL

In Newfoundland evaluation of the Project will be done in two stages. Stage one will be primarily formative: An implementation analysis will be conducted to document the steps required to initiate the Project, and a process evaluation will describe the Project at all stages. In stage two, an impact or summative assessment will be conducted to determine whether the Project is meeting its goals. Together, these will allow for comparison of the actual Project to what had been envisioned by the planners. A number of process evaluations have been done in similar projects (e.g., Chambers, 1979; Charney & Kiteman, 1971; Kviz, Misener, & Vinson, 1983), as have a number of impact assessments (e.g., Chambers, Bruce-Lockhert, Black, Sampson, & Burte, 1977; Spitzer et al., 1974). However, the present project differs in that one of its goals is to involve the community in the public health care process.

Stage 1: Success in the first year will depend on more than the motivation of the planners and nurses: people in key positions in the government and community, as well as local residents, will also need to be convinced of the importance of the Project and its benefits. Thus, the influence of these people on the Project must be investigated. The methods used during Stage 1 will be a combination of the naturalistic approach described by Guba and Lincoln (1981) and the qualitative method described by Patton (1980), which allow for exploratory responses rather than multiple-choice alternatives. These methods include interviews, participant observation, and examination of records and archival material, and will provide the information to interpret the influence that different groups are having on the Project.

At the end of this stage it will be possible to compare the actual Project with what was proposed, and the this assessment will determine whether to go on to Stage 2.

If operations conform to what has been proposed, then the Project is likely innovative, and a summative/impact assessment should be undertaken next. On the other hand, if the Project has succumbed to traditional demands (e. g., nurses find themselves primarily delivering home care instead of involving the community in the public health care process), it could not be considered novel, and there may be no reason for further assessment.

Stage 2: The impact assessment will involve collecting information to examine whether the Project is achieving its goals. There are three parties involved in this evaluation, each emphasizing slightly different goals. The Association of Registered Nurses of Newfoundland and the Danish Nurses Organization will want to know if the Project is meeting the 12 goals stated in the proposal, while governing bodies in Canada and Denmark will want to know if the project is effecting a measurable improvement in health status and if it is cost-effective. In addition, the Canadian government will want to know if the Project is managing to involve the community in all aspects of program planning.

The measurement of health status will focus on outcome indices. Traditionally, health status outcomes have measured negative indicators, focusing more on illness than health (Hargart & Billington, 1982; Parker, 1983; Sackett, Chambers, MacPherson, Goldsmith, & Maculey, 1977), but both positive and negative measures will be incorporated here. The indicators selected for measurement are: pregnancy outcomes, child nutrition, immunizations, infection incidence, recurrent complaints, hospital admission, deaths, adult obesity, and prevalence of hypertension. It is expected that evaluation of the Project will be funded for only three years, which is too short a period to find actual changes in many of these outcome measures; therefore, information related to lifestyle over this period will also be collected. There is evidence that modifications in lifestyle may take less time to achieve and (assuming that they are sustained) may have long-term health consequences, for example, reduction in smoking.

On the surface the cost component of the equation appears to be relatively simple: an additive process of accumulating all the costs related to nurses' salaries and travel, clinic expenses, and other direct disbursals. However, indirect costs also come into play, such as referrals to physicians or hospital emergency departments, and tests and procedures related to these referrals. These indirect costs may, however, be quite necessary and may, in fact, lead to reduced future costs because of early detection of potential debilitating disease and, therefore, reduced morbidity.

While cost determination may be difficult, net benefits may be even more elusive. When dealing with return on each invested "health care" dollar, the returns are multifaceted whether short- or long-term. Furthermore, the measures used may be difficult and "soft" in nature. How much is saved, for example, by providing extensive home care services to the elderly (current dollars) with the objective of keeping them out of expensive nursing homes (future dollars) as long as possible?

In addition, unlike business, which uses basically one measure in a relatively closed system, the health care system uses many measures in an open system with a great deal of "leakage." Some people within the selected communities may circumvent the system by accessing health care resources at a different location. For example, most cottage hospitals in Newfoundland experienced a significant decline in deliveries when transportation improved and specialists were available in major centers.

To simplify the effort, three or four outcome criteria will be chosen early in the process as indications of benefits, rather than an attempt made to cover all possible outcomes. The choice of these criteria will be made in collaboration with the ARNN and the evaluation team in Denmark. These criteria might be as simple as a head count of the number of people accessing the health care system through the nurses at the primary care level, or as complex as a measure of the general health status of the community. (These decisions will be made only after the practice has started.) Finally, health status, lifestyle, and cost outcomes will be evaluated by comparing conditions in the practice region before and after the start of the Practice, and against one or two control communities.

In summary, the formative evaluation will determine if the Project is innovative, and the summative evaluation will determine the economic feasibility of this nursing model and whether it can be generalized to larger populations.

EVALUATION AT THE PRACTICE LEVEL

As previously mentioned, all Practice nursing personnel will be required to use standard assessment tools and recording systems. Primary nurses will be held accountable for the outcomes of care for all clients in their caseloads. Concurrent and retroactive record audits will be carried out by nursing staff, through methods that have been specifically designed for the Practice. Over time, their application and the comparison of their results to accepted standards of care and to desirable outcomes, as jointly determined by the primary nurse and the client, should provide an accurate evaluation of the effectiveness of interventions. Further, it should be possible to link specific interventions to specific needs.

This kind of evaluation is relatively new in nursing, and it is hoped that it will contribute to the small but growing body of knowledge in nursing diagnoses and treatment. Linkage with a joint European-WHO study on quality assurance nursing has already been initiated and will be followed up in the Practice setting.

References

Chambers, L. W., Bruce-Lockhert, P., Black, D., Sampson, E., & Burte, M. (1977). A controlled trial of the impact family practice nurse on volume, quality and cost of rural health services. *Medical Care, 15*(12), 971-981.

Chambers, L. W. (1979). Financial impact on family practice. Nurses on medical practice in Canada. *Inquiry, 15*(4), 339-349.

Charney, E., & Kiteman, H. (1971). The child-health nurse (pediatric nurse practitioner) in private practice: A controlled trial. *New England Journal of Medicine, 295,* 1353-1358.

Guba, E. G., & Lincoln, Y. S. (1981). *Effective evaluations*. San Francisco: Jossey-Bass.

Hargart, J., & Billington, D. R. (1982). Towards an understanding of health status: The perceived importance of health status dimensions. *Community Medicine, 4*, 12-24.

Kviz, F. J., Misener, T. R., & Vinson, N. (1983). Rural health care: Consumers' perceptions of nurse practitioner role. *Journal of Community Health, 8*(4), 248-262.

Mahler, H. (1985). *Nurses lead the way*. (WHO Features). Geneva, Switzerland: WHO.

Parker, S. O. (1983). A conceptual model for outcome assessment. *Nurse Practitioner, 8*(1), 41, 44-45.

Patton, M. Q. (1980). *Qualitative evaluating methods*. Beverly Hills, CA: Sage.

Sackett, D. L., Chambers, L. W., MacPherson, A. S., Goldsmith, C. H., & Maculey, R. G. (1977). The development and appreciation of indices of health: General methods and a summary of results. *American Journal of Public Health, 67*(5), 423-428.

Spitzer, W. O., Sackett, D. L., Sibley, J. C., Roberts, R. S., Gent, M., Kergin, D. J., Hackett, B. C., & Olynich, A. (1974). The Burlington randomized trial of the nurse practitioner. *New England Journal of Medicine, 290*, 251-256.

World Health Organization. (1984). *Organization of primary health care in communities* (SHS/IAH/84.1). Geneva: WHO.

14 What Does the Primary Care Physician Do in Patient Care That Makes a Difference? Five Approaches to One Question

MARTIN J. BASS
HOWARD BRODY
CECIL G. HELMAN
JOHN G. R. HOWIE
HENK LAMBERTS
PETER G. NORTON
BARBARA STARFIELD

As a final topic for this volume, Martin Bass posed a question: "What does the primary care physician do in patient care that makes a difference?" Drs. Starfield, Brody, Helman, Lamberts, and Howie each agreed to formulate a research agenda around this question.

Their responses, which follow, are what one would expect: individual, perceptive, insightful, and innovative. Dr. Starfield, an epidemiologist, presents a summary of her generic approach to any research question, and then highlights this approach by considering aspects of the posed question. She focuses on the issues of question, population, hypothesis, measures, and interpretation. Dr. Brody, a philosopher as well as a clinician, grapples with the meaning of the question itself. He models for the reader the necessary steps for creation of a research question from a general question, such as the one posed here, and struggles to link his convictions about the meaning and goals of primary care with his recent readings. Through this process, he emerges with a brilliant primary care research question. Dr. Helman, an anthropologist and a clinician, invites us to consider the question from three patient and physician viewpoints (a "triplopia"): attitudes, behaviors, and physiology. Dr. Lamberts (1987), a clinician and director of a multipractice registration study in the Netherlands (the Transition Project), explains how the database that resulted from his project could be used and enhanced to answer the question. His approach is to examine the intersection of patient values and doctor norms by assessing the main reasons for encounter as viewed by each party.

Finally, Dr. Howie, an academic family physician, stresses that a research question must be, as well as answerable, interesting and important to the investigator. In particular, he cautions that the appropriate tools must either be available or be developed. He translates the general question to a specific one that is different from any that the others posed.

These five responses can serve as role models for us by displaying different and diverse specific questions, research methods, and acceptable standards. It could be argued that to answer such a question, one that is central to primary care, multiple specific questions must be addressed and that each question may need its own methods and standards.

DR. BARBARA STARFIELD: What I am going to do is explain five principles that guide me in my own research and in research consultation.

The first point, regardless of whether a question is my own or somebody else's, is why in the world is the question being asked? Let us take the proposed question in particular: "What does the primary care physician do in patient care that makes a difference?" There are many reasons why this question may have been posed. Let us suppose the reason is that we feel defensive, are concerned about future funding for primary care, and want to set up a study that will influence the people who are responsible for policy decisions. As you can see, you really have to be clear why you are asking the question in order to narrow the framework for the study.

The second point is to consider what the question is really about, what is implied about the population that will be studied. You have to get a clear understanding of the definition of the proposed study population.

The third component is the hypothesis. In research it is not always necessary to have a hypothesis; rather, it is possible to conduct studies whose aim is to *generate* hypotheses. However, if a proposed study does have a hypothesis, it must be out in the open, since its statement will help decide what variables need to be in the equations and what data will be collected.

The fourth thing to be considered is the data source: Do you have access to the data, or must you collect it? If some of the data needed are not available (e.g., you cannot recruit patients), then you will not be able to answer even the best posed question. Consider the specific question again: What does a primary care physician do in patient care that makes a difference? The operational terms here (the variables) are *do* and *difference.* What is meant by "do"—what kind of things are included? Is the important thing problem recognition, diagnosis, therapy, reassessment, or something in another framework? The researcher has to consider the question, "What do you mean by 'do'?" It is the same thing with "difference"—what kind of things are you going to consider important in making a difference?

Going back to the general case, you must also consider what things you will be able to measure. Limitations include your skills, the instruments at hand, and available resource people. Similar limitations apply to eventual analysis: If you have only certain skills yourself, or if only certain skills are available to you, there is no point in setting up a design that you just cannot deal with.

The fifth and final point centers on the interpretation. This brings us full circle and back to the question. What kinds of interpretations are you going to be willing to put on your data? Are there certain findings that would be so unacceptable that you would not be willing to spend time and energy on a study that might reveal these findings? I think this is a very important consideration.

These five points are a framework that I would use in considering this question or in counseling somebody who proposed it.

DR. HOWARD BRODY: I cannot reply to the question as it was posed, because I think I know the answer. I will, however, at the end of my remarks, discuss a related question that could be researched. I think it interesting that, since I think I know the answer to the posed question, if someone did a research project and got a different answer, I probably would not believe it. I am going to tell you what I think the answer is, rather than describe how I would do the research project.

One attractive answer to this question, what does a family doctor do in patient care that makes a difference, was provided by John Berger in the book, *A Fortunate Man*(1976). There were two things in this book that, to me, seem to describe this: *recognizing* and being the *clerk of records*.

Recognizing is a technical term that Berger, a sociologist, defines as follows: Anguished patients (not just sick, but truly anguished) are somehow convinced that they are no longer part of the human community. They feel that their illness has made them so different that they are not recognizable as people. They come to the physician, offering their illness, fully convinced that they cannot be recognized as people anymore, but hoping that at least their illness might be recognized. Berger says that recognition has occurred when the family physician succeeds in meeting this expectation. In doing so the doctor reestablishes the bridge of humanity, and the patient once more feels part of the human community. In essence, the physician reaches out to the patient and says, "I recognize what is human in you, that you have been so anguished about the illness that you have forgotten that humanity is still there in you. My humanity reaches out and recognizes the humanity that you still have."

The *clerk of the records* concept describes how the physician engages in the conversation of the community at a pub or local gatherings. This idea centers around the importance of the physician as one who validates communal knowledge and memory. Berger observes that many conversations between physicians and patients begin with "do you remember when?" The scientifically trained physician, as a member of the community, validates everyone else's memories and confirms, "Yes, it did happen that way." This is, however, a very humble role; the physician is not an archbishop but merely a clerk of the records, invited in only at the will of the members of the community to carry out the humble but important function of validating their records.

It is interesting to look at these two functions for two reasons. First, they are both social bridging functions, and second, the themes that run through both of them are wholeness and coherence. Because they involve these reasons, I find them attractive answers to the question of what do we family physicians do that is important.

I have recently been trying to incorporate these concepts into my work and have developed a framework that I call the joint construction of narrative. The model claims that the generic feature of a patient's presenting complaint is, "My story is broken. Can you help me fix it?" Usually there is more: "I think I have a story, but it scares me and I do not like it. The story that I am telling myself is a dysfunctional one and I can't live comfortably with it. Doctor, help me construct a better story that will cause me less discomfort and distress." In an extreme case the patient might mean: "I cannot tell myself a story." My concept is that the family physician has to listen carefully enough to know the patient's story and determine whether it is functional or not from the patient's perspective; and then, using medical knowledge and models of prevention and treatment, help construct a new story that is recognized and can be owned by the patient.

That was what I thought the answer was when I came to cooperate on this book. But, I must confess that I am a bit puzzled. My puzzlement has arisen from a number of things that I was either reminded of by the other chapters or read here for the first time. One thing that struck me was Donna Manca's paper on women's accounts of their miscarriages (Chapter 11). The qualitative design got at the experience of miscarriage and its value to women: what was good, what was healing, and so on. One woman's comment to the interviewer was very revealing to me: "This was the first time I have had a chance to tell my whole story. Other people have asked me for specific pieces of my story, based on what they were concerned with, but this is the first time I have had a chance to tell the whole story" (Manca, 1989).

Thinking about this has led me to be more humble. I might have to give up the idea of the joint construction of narrative. I wonder if what attracted me to it was physician activism.

Let me hypothesize a new model. Doctors like to think they are doing something. In a consultation, the important thing is that the doctor listens and the listening is what really does the work. If the doctor "fixes the narrative" later, it might be that the patient gives it back to make the doctor feel good. What really was therapeutic, what really made a difference, was the listening to the story.

That is, to me, the interesting research question. Of course, the answer could be a bit of both my old idea and my new model. In the short run what I do that makes a difference is to listen to the story. However, in the long run what I might do is help fix the story. That is my hunch and that is my research agenda.

DR. CECIL HELMAN: One of my ideas has already been discussed by Dr. Brody. As an anthropologist, I was going to say that the important thing is that family physicians are healers. It is interesting to compare family physicians to other healers in other locations: in other cultures, in hospitals, in the community, and so on.

Healers in all cultures and backgrounds have certain things in common. While they heal the body, mind, and spirit, they also do something more subtle and hidden. They try to put Humpty Dumpty together again. (This is similar to what Dr. Brody has written.) They reassemble the patient's worldview.

Ill health, particularly an acute event, results in physical and psychological symptoms for the patient. But more happens. The continuity and the coherence of the patient's world are shattered for a moment. When a healer listens to the narrative story, the patient's tale is reestablished as part of the bigger story of the world. Healers try to fit the individual's suffering into a wider framework.

Starting from this perspective, one can develop a research agenda for family medicine. The agenda requires that we develop a "triplopia," which involves looking simultaneously at three things. First, we must examine attitudes, beliefs, and narratives in order to understand both what people think and what they say they think. Second, we must look at behavior, either self-reported or observed. Third, we must consider the physiology: what the body says.

This "triplopia" leads to three conceptual views of the patient, each of which may be entirely incompatible with the others. The attitudes, behaviors, and physiology of a patient may run on three different tracks. For example, you could have 10 people all drinking the same amount of beer every day, and yet their individual physiologies might be quite different. So one has to have the conception of multiple perspectives converging on any particular case.

I would also suggest that the research issue include the doctor; that is, that the attitudes, behavior, and physiology of the doctor be studied as well. One must question whether he or she puts together the world—reassembles Humpty Dumpty—during the consultation. In fact, maybe the whole aim of being a doctor or a healer is an attempt to reassemble the shattered Humpty Dumpty within oneself.

I make an appeal. By all means use social science along with quantitative physiological techniques, but move the doctor into the framework with the patient. This will lead to a "reflexive" approach, which is one of the contributions of feminist anthropology. It can be described as dropping the mask—the bogus mask—of objectivity, and being more involved in the situation: admitting one's influences upon it and vice versa.

I will cite one personal example where my research project influenced me (Helman, 1981): where the attitudes, beliefs, and behavior of a group of people whom I studied affected my own attitudes, beliefs, and behavior. Some years ago I interviewed 50 people, both men and women, mostly middle-aged, all of whom had been taking benzodiazepines for a minimum of six months. Conventionally, these subjects would be considered to be "hooked" on their drugs. Every month, regular as clockwork, all 50 would attend their doctors to get their prescriptions renewed for enormous amounts of Valium or Nitrazepam.

When I studied these people, all of whom were being treated exactly the same by their doctors, I found three different metaphors that they used to describe their drug use.

One group saw the drug as a tonic, in that they took it only occasionally and had control over it. These patients would say, "Well, when I need a tonic, I take it. When I feel tense, I take it."

The second group used it as a type of fuel, feeling that without the drug, they wouldn't function in a social way. These people saw themselves as essentially "bad," but with their medication, they were able to fulfill social expectations. This finding was similar to that of the late Ruth Cooperstock (1979) of the Addiction Research Foundation in Toronto. In her study, most of the subjects who were addicted to Valium were women. These women told her, "Without Valium, I am a very irritable and unhappy person. However, with it, I am a nurturing person, a very nice person, and so on."

The third group saw the drug as a food. They were, in the main, elderly. Their view was that without the drug, not only would they be unable to function socially, but they would actually die.

This study influenced my behavior. I understood that, contrary to their physicians' opinions, patients "hooked" on benzodiazepines are not a homogeneous group. I thought that a doctor might be able to tailor the treatment to individual patients. For example, if a patient viewed the drug as a tonic, then it would not be necessary to prescribe a large amount every month. The patient should be encouraged to use the medication only when it was needed. In fact, all patients should be counseled to move toward the tonic end of the spectrum.

In contrast, the group who saw themselves essentially as bad people, who could only fulfill social expectations if they used the drug, would need a different approach. In particular, they should respond to therapy designed to enhance a stronger vision of themselves and their positions in the world.

The third group, who saw Valium as a food, would be the most difficult of all. One would have to nourish them in another way. These people often felt that, with the drug in their house, they were not alone. They were socially isolated, so tailoring the treatment to them meant trying to break their isolation.

The important research efforts in the future will thus try to unravel patients' and doctors' beliefs and behaviors. The findings will lead to improvements in the way doctors deal with people.

DR. HENK LAMBERTS: I begin with the idea that there is a difference between the subjective values of patients; the more objective, normative approaches of doctors; and the collective norms of society. I would focus on this margin between the values of patients and the norms of doctors, and consider a number of aspects of function: physical, psychological, and social.

I would attempt to ascertain what doctors *really* do for 1,000 patients per year. That is my unknown, and to go on, I would have to know that data. To reliably determine these data, I would set up a routine database that included complete episodes and measures of functional status as seen and assessed by the patient and by the family physician. I would measure it (functional status) objectively, using the COOP charts (Lamberts, 1990).

I would first examine this database by looking for discrepancies: Where do the patient and the doctor disagree? Then I would examine how function changes over time and over episodes, what daily activities are limited in each patient, and the physical and emotional condition of the patient at each consultation. If the patients were suffering pain, I would grade the severity. Finally, I would like to know what patients think about changes in their function and health, and what the doctors think about such changes.

Using this database I would exclude those episodes that had an acute course over time. From the Transition Project, it is known that 50% of new episodes are over with in four weeks (are acute). I would focus on subacute (taking one to six months to resolve) or chronic episodes, so there would be enough time to see whether the doctor's intervention makes a difference. The distribution of the conditions (demographics, diagnosis, symptoms, and so forth) for these longer episodes would be determined, to see if it was the same as that seen in the Transition Project, in order to establish a reference point.

I would probably limit my study to patients 65 years and over. Older patients have many psychological and social problems in addition to their chronic and subacute conditions, and I believe that this combination makes this group one in which family physicians can make the most difference.

For the study population, it would be important to determine the reasons for encounter (RFE). In particular:

• how often such patients initiate an episode with a psychological or social complaint;

• how often the doctor initiates an episode with the reason for encounter being a psychological or social problem.

As an illustration, I hypothesize that family physicians are extremely effective with one subgroup of the study population: those patients presenting with the fear of cancer (or another disease of perceived similar seriousness). In the Transition Project, 9% of patients presented with this complaint in the registration year.

In summary, to study the proposed problem I would work with an ICPC episode-oriented database, with patient- and doctor-evaluated function status added to it. I would concentrate on longer episodes, so that there was time to see important changes that might be attributable to the doctor's intervention. To measure which changes are important, I would use both the doctor and the patient as judges. Routine databases would only elucidate one part of the picture, and I would need specific studies to complement it.

DR. JOHN HOWIE: There is a little fishing village called Cruden Bay, about 20 miles north of Aberdeen. Just south of Cruden Bay there is a crossroads sign, which reads: "Cruden Bay, 5 miles this way," and "Cruden Bay, 5 miles that way." The story is told of an American visitor who had arrived and found himself perplexed at the choice available to him. He asked a passing farm laborer, "Say, my good man, does it matter which way I go to Cruden Bay?" To which the answer was, "Nae to me."

And to me the answer to the question is: "Nae to me." I am afraid it doesn't appeal to me very much. If I were to consider the problem by looking at principles, I would go back to my two sets of principles about interesting and important events. I would have to say that the question, as it is worded, is not interesting or important to me, and so I would begin by negotiating a more specific question.

I have, by focusing down, managed to persuade myself that the question is potentially interesting and important. In this I have something in common with Dr. Lamberts. I feel that he has discussed almost all points that I wanted to consider. However, I have narrowed down to one single thing which he did not consider and which, if true, would satisfy me with respect to the question "what do family doctors do that makes a difference?"

Not surprisingly, I have focused on the question: "during consultation, does the doctor improve the state of psychosocial well-being of the patient?" I assume that the answer is yes. As a secondary question I am going to ask, "Do quick doctors, as defined in my chapter (Chapter 2), do it less well than slow doctors?" I admit that you could also ask, "Do doctors do it better than nurses? Do nurses do it better than receptionists?" There is a whole variety of related questions.

The question in this form is interesting, important, and answerable. But there is one more of my principles that the question (now rephrased) needs to meet. Can we identify an accessible and definable numerator and an accessible and definable denominator?

The Nottingham Health Profile (Kind & Carr-Hill, 1987) is a self-administered health status measure comprised of two measures of physical health and pain and four of psychological and social health. It has been validated in England, and I assume (this may be questioned) that it is therefore valid in Scotland as well. (There is always a risk in trying to translate a measure from one country to another: The measure may lose some refinement of meaning, and that may make it less acceptable and useful.) I would administer it to patients before they have a consultation and again a month after, to see whether their response had improved. I have narrowed Dr. Bass's question down to a measurement of this effect. In fact, our research group has already started this study, and you will know the answer in the near future. What we have found so far is that about 30% of patients who consult us in our inner-city disadvantaged practice have important psychological or social problems we have missed or have not had time to address.

DR. PETER NORTON: So there you have it. Five different but complementary approaches to the same question. The original question is central to primary care research but was too general, so each of the writers has rephrased it to suit his or her research agenda and concept of primary care. I think questions such as the one Dr. Bass posed are best attacked by breaking them into researchable pieces. Each piece may require a different research method, and each method will have its own standards and protocols. Some of these methods and standards exist, others will be borrowed from other branches of science, and still others will need to be created as our discipline matures. The use of multiple approaches will be complementary to our practice and the resulting research agenda will help us deliver better and more comprehensive care to our patients.

If we carefully examine the responses to the question proposed above, two factors are apparent. First, each contributor rephrased and focused the question so that it was "owned" and thus became a question to which the investigator could be committed. Second, each contributor has suggested a research method that relied on his or her own individual expertise and experience.

We are generalists, and practice in that condition. We must allow our generalist skills to carry over into our research agenda. We must use the expertise and sophistication of our specialist colleagues, whether in medicine, social science, behavioral science, or any other research discipline, and adapt them with their standards to our unique and important field. This book has attempted to facilitate this vision, and we hope that it will aid and assist all researchers in their attempts to better understand the primary care interface and improve it.

References

Berger, J., & Mohr, J. (1976). *A fortunate man*. London: Writers and Readers Publishing Co-operative.

Cooperstock, R. (1979). A review of women's psychotropic drug use. *Canadian Journal of Psychiatry, 24*(1), 29-34.

Helman, C. G. (1981). "Tonic," "Fuel" and "Food": Social and symbolic aspects of long-term use of psychotropic drugs. *Social Science and Medicine, 15B*, 521-533.

Kind, P., & Carr-Hill, R. (1987). The Nottingham Health Profile: A useful tool for epidemiologists? *Social Sciences and Medicine, 25*(8), 905-910.

Lamberts, H. (1990). The use of functional status assessment within the framework of the International Classification of Primary Care. In J. Froom (Ed.), *Functional status measurement in primary care*. New York: Springer-Verlag.

Lamberts, H., Brouwer, H., Groen, A. S. M., & Huisman, H. (1987). Het transitiemodel in de huisartspraktijk. Praktisch gebruik van de ICPC tijdens 28.000 contacten. *Huisarts en Wetenschap, 30*, 105-113.

Manca, D. (1989, February). *Study of miscarriage through qualitative and quantitative methods*. Paper presented at the Conference on Basic Sciences of Primary Care Research, Toronto, Canada.

Index

About the Authors

Martin J. Bass, MD, MSc, CCFP, FCFP, is Director of the Centre for Studies in Family Medicine at The University of Western Ontario, London, Ontario, Canada. He is a Professor of Family Medicine and Epidemiology and is a practicing family physician. He was the sole Canadian and the only family physician to be appointed as one of 29 Kellogg International Fellows. His research expertise includes hypertension in family practice, natural history of headaches, technology application in family practice, prevention, and quality of care.

Howard Brody, MD, Ph.D., is Associate Professor of Family Practice and Philosophy, and Director of the Center for Ethics and Humanities in the Life Sciences, at Michigan State University, East Lansing, Michigan. His primary areas of research and teaching have been medical ethics and philosophy of medicine.

Judith Belle Brown, Ph.D., is an Assistant Professor in the Department of Family Medicine at The University of Western Ontario, London, Ontario, Canada. With teaching and research interests in doctor-patient communication, she has presented local and national workshops to residents and faculty, and has been published in such journals as *Family Practice: An International Journal, Canadian Medical Association Journal,* and the *Canadian Family Physician.* She received her Ph.D. from Smith College.

Benjamin F. Crabtree, Ph.D., is Assistant Professor of Family Medicine and Anthropology at the University of Connecticut, Hartford, Connecticut. A medical anthropologist with wide-ranging experience, he has served with the Peace Corps in Ethiopia as a Surveillance Officer in the World Health Organization's Smallpox Eradication Program, and in Korea, where he assisted and trained health personnel in a remote mountain district for the Korean National Tuberculosis Association. While in Korea he completed a study exploring the relationship between socioeconomic/educational status and birth outcomes. He is currently the Associate Director of Research in the Department of Family Medicine, and has recently serve as Director of the Research Curriculum for the Travelers' Center on Aging Geriatric Fellowship Program. With Dr. Miller, he is spearheading a national effort to incorporate a better balance of methodologies in North American primary health care research.

Robert A. Cushman, MD, is Assistant Professor of Family Medicine at the University of Connecticut School of Medicine, Hartford, Connecticut. He completed his undergraduate degree at Amherst College in 1976, then continued research in cell biology for three years before proceeding to Emory University School of Medicine, receiving his MD in 1983. His postgraduate training in family medicine was at the Highland Hospital/University of Rochester program and included an extra year serving as co-chief resident and pursuing additional training in family therapy. His research interests include family systems and health, specifically the relationship of family/social support and decisions about nursing home admissions for the elderly; exploring qualitative research methods for primary care research; and improving techniques for medical education and patient education.

Earl V. Dunn, MD, FCFP(C), has been a Professor in the Department of Family and Community Medicine since 1982, and is also a Professor at the Centre for Studies in Medical Education at the University of Toronto, Toronto, Ontario, Canada. Born in the Province of Quebec in 1931, Dr. Dunn was educated in Quebec and New Brunswick and graduated from McGill University Medical School in 1960. He did a two-year general practice residency in Kansas City, Missouri, and then entered practice in a mining community in the Province of Quebec. In 1968 he became a full-time member of the Faculty of Medicine, University of Toronto. Dr. Dunn has specific research interests in medical decision making, telemedicine, resource utilization, and the economics of health care delivery. He has also published in all these fields.

Dana Edge, RN, MSN, earned her BSN from the University of Iowa and an MSN in Primary Care from the University of North Carolina at Chapel Hill. She has practiced as a staff nurse in various settings and continues to practice as a Regional Relief Nurse in Labrador. Since 1986 she has coordinated the Community and Primary Health Care Nursing Program at the School of Nursing, Memorial University of Newfoundland. Primary health care and the health of aboriginal peoples remain her major research interests.

Toula M. Gerace, RN, BScN, is a Clinical Lecturer in the Department of Family Medicine at The University of Western Ontario, London, Ontario, Canada. With clinical and research interests in health promotion, disease prevention, and a special interest in the area of collaboration, she has presented workshops and research findings at local and national meetings. She has been published in such journals as *Family Medicine,* the *Journal of Medical Education,* and the *Canadian Family Physician.*

Dorothy C. Hall, RN, was educated in Canada and the United States. Her experience in the field of health care has included work in Outpost Nursing Stations in Northern Canada, teaching in schools and faculties of nursing, and the administration of hospital nursing services. For 26 years she worked for the World Health Organization (WHO) in field and regional office positions in both the Southeast Asia and European Regions of WHO. She is the author of numerous papers and articles dealing with health and nursing and is currently the International Coordinator for the Danish-Canadian (Newfoundland) Project, Primary Health Care—A Nursing Model.

Cecil G. Helman, MB, ChB, MRCGP, Diplomate Soc. Anthro., was born in Cape Town, South Africa, graduated from the

University of Cape Town Medical School in 1967, and has lived in London, England, since 1969. In 1972 he graduated in social anthropology from University College, University of London, and then went into family practice on the outskirts of London. In 1983-1984 he was Visiting Fellow in Social Medicine and Health Policy, and Visiting Scholar in Primary Care at Harvard Medical School. Since 1984 he has been a Lecturer in the Department of Primary Health Care, University College and Middlesex Medical School, and Research Fellow, Department of Anthropology, University College, London. His areas of research have included lay health beliefs and their relation to medical treatment; doctor-patient communication; symbolic aspects of psychotropic drug use; psychosomatic disorders; cultural and social aspects of heart disease; and the role of cultural factors in health, disease, and medical care. He teaches medical anthropology to medical students, residents, family physicians, nurses, and other health professionals and also conducts short courses on cross-cultural health care. Dr. Helman has been a visiting guest lecturer at many universities and medical schools in Britain, Europe, and North America. In addition to papers on medical anthropology, the second edition of his textbook, *Culture, Health and Illness: An Introduction for Health Professionals,* was published in 1990.

John G. R. Howie, MD, Ph.D., FRCPE, FRCGP, is Professor of General Practice at the University of Edinburgh, Edinburgh, Scotland. After four years in laboratory medicine, he entered general practice in 1966, working first in "full-time" in Glasgow. Subsequently he was Lecturer and later Senior Lecturer in General Practice in Aberdeen. Since 1960 he has been Professor of General Practice in Edinburgh. His research interests have included studies of how General Practitioners use antibiotics and, more recently, how they arrange their work and the stresses related to it. He is the author of *Research in General Practice,* the second edition of which was published in 1989.

Anton J. Kuzel, MD, MHPE, is Associate Professor, Department of Family Practice, at the Medical College of Virginia, Virginia Commonwealth University, Fairfax, Virginia. Having completed his undergraduate, graduate, and postgraduate training at the

University of Illinois, Dr. Kuzel has served as Associate Director of the Fairfax Family Practice Program in Fairfax, Virginia, and is now Coordinator of Graduate Programs and Faculty Development in the Department of Family Practice at MCV-VCU in Richmond, Virginia. His research interests include the practical application of qualitative inquiry to family medicine research, with particular emphasis on the doctor-patient relationship, preventive care, and chemical dependency.

Henk Lamberts, MD, Ph.D., has been Professor and Chairman of the Department of Family Medicine, at the University of Amsterdam, Amsterdam, The Netherlands, since 1984. He attended the Medical School at the University of Utrecht and the Medical School of Rotterdam. He did his thesis at Leiden University. In 1972 he founded the Ommoord Health Centre in Rotterdam. From 1976 to 1984 he was an active general practitioner. Dr. Lamberts is actively engaged in the development of the International Classification of Health Problems in Primary Care, of Inclusion Criteria for its main rubrics (ICHPPC-2-Defined), and of the International Classification of Process in Primary Care (IC-Process-PC). Together with Professor Maurice Wood, he is editor of the new International Classification of Primary Care (ICPC) and is project leader of the ICPC project in the European Community. Dr. Lamberts is responsible for the Transition Project of the University of Amsterdam, which concentrates on the construction of a detailed and reliable episode-oriented epidemiology of family medicine. On this basis, tools to register and classify patient data are being developed and tested.

Robert C. Like, MD, MS, is Assistant Professor in the Department of Family Medicine of the University of Medicine and Dentistry of New Jersey (UMDNJ), Robert Wood Johnson Medical School, New Brunswick, New Jersey. Dr. Like graduated from Dartmouth College with a BA in Anthropology in 1974, and received his MD from Harvard Medical School in 1979. He served his postgraduate family practice residency training at the University Hospitals of Cleveland (Ohio) and earned an MS in Family Medicine in a Robert Wood Johnson Academic Family Medicine Fellowship at Case Western Reserve University, also in Cleveland. He is a board-certified family physician and a member of the American Academy of Family Physicians, the Society of Teachers of Family Medicine, and the North American Primary Care Research Group. Dr. Like combines a busy clinical practice with a variety of administrative, educational, and research responsibilities. He is also a member of the Developmental Grants Review Subcommittee of the Agency for Health Care Policy and Research (formerly NCHSR). His research interests include health services utilization by adults with chronic disabilities; small area variation in medical outcomes and procedures; the doctor-patient relationship in primary care; and clinically applied anthropology.

Ian R. McWhinney, MD, is Professor, Department of Family Medicine at The University of Western Ontario, London, Ontario, Canada. He received his medical degree from Cambridge University in 1949 and spent 14 years in general practice in England before coming to Western in 1968. His interests include the philosophy and history of medicine, the diagnostic process, and the natural history of disease. He has been published on these subjects in the *Lancet*, the *New England Journal of Medicine*, the *Canadian Medical Association Journal*, the *Proceedings of the Royal Society of Medicine*, the *Journal of Medicine and Philosophy*, the *Journal of Medical Education*, and the *Journal of Family Practice*. His textbook of family medicine was published in 1989.

Donna Patricia Manca, BMSc, MD, CCFP, MClSc, is an Assistant Professor of Family Medicine at the University of Alberta, Edmonton, Alberta, Canada, and has a teaching practice at the Family Clinic in Edmonton. She earned her BMSc and graduated from Medicine at the University of Alberta. She completed a thesis on *The Miscarriage Experience*, with the help of Dr. Martin Bass as her chief adviser. The thesis was successfully defended, contributing to her being awarded an MClSc in 1988.

William L. Miller, MD, MA, is Assistant Professor of Family Medicine and Anthropology at the University of Connecticut, Hartford, Connecticut. He graduated from Wake Forest University with honors and received an MA in Medical Anthropology. During two years as a secondary school teacher in the Caribbean, he also completed ethnographic fieldwork investigating psychosocial aspects of hypertension in the Bay Islands of Honduras, followed by a quantitative and qualitative investigation of psychosocial and nutritional aspects of hypertension on Saba Island. He then pursued his medical training at the University of North Carolina School of Medicine, receiving his MD in 1977. After completing a family practice residency at Harrisburg Hospital, where he served as co-chief resident, he was in private practice in Bethlehem, Pennsylvania, for four years. Dr. Miller's clinical and research interests are in healing, hypertension, family systems and family theory, medical anthropology, the doctor-patient relationship, and multimethod research strategies.

Brian A. P. Morris, MD, CCFP, FCFP(C), is Assistant Professor in the Department of Family and Community Medicine at the University of Toronto, Toronto, Ontario, Canada. A Fellow of the College of Family Physicians of Canada, Dr. Morris graduated from the University of Toronto in 1978. Following two years of family practice residency at St. Michael's Hospital in Toronto, he established his practice in the small city of Barrie, Ontario. Although his research has developed fairly recently, Dr. Morris is the author of more than 20 published papers. Three of the early papers were case reports, leading to his current interest in the methodology and style of case reporting. He also has a full-time teaching practice linked with the University of Toronto.

Peter G. Norton, BSc, MA, Ph.D., MD, CCFP, is an Associate Professor in the Department of Family and Community Medicine at the University of Toronto and also Chairman of the Department of Family and Community Medicine at the Sunnybrook Health Science Centre, Toronto, Ontario, Canada. He came late to family medicine after a first career in mathematics. Following his family medicine training, he joined the staff of the University of Toronto and helped found the Primary Care Research Unit at Sunnybrook Health Science Centre, a teaching complex owned by the university. His research interests include medical decision making, utilization of health care resources, alternative models of health care delivery, and research methodologies for primary care.

Garfield A. Pynn, BComm, MBA, is Director of the P. J. Gardiner Institute for Small Business Studies and is a member of the Faculty of Business, Memorial University of Newfoundland, St. John's, Newfoundland, Canada. An adviser on policy, operations, and program development for several provincial governments, national research and educational institutions, and national and international business organizations, Mr. Pynn served on the Royal Commission on Hospital and Home Costs in Newfoundland during 1983 and 1984. This Commission's major report, on the cost of providing health care within the hospital and nursing homes systems in the Province, was positively endorsed by virtually all segments within this complex environment and has served as a business plan for the Provincial government in planning for the 1990s. He is currently a Director of the St. John's Home Care Program, which administers the provision of Acute and Continuing Care, and Home Support programs to the local community. Mr. Pynn's research on small business has been published in the proceedings of several World Conferences on Small Business, in the *Journal of Small Business-Canada*, and in the *Journal of Small Business Management*.

Abraham S. Ross, Ph.D., heads the Department of Psychology at the Memorial University of Newfoundland, St. John's, Newfoundland, Canada. Dr. Ross has taught courses in program evaluation at the graduate and undergraduate level and has conducted evaluations for the federal and provincial governments.

Barbara Starfield, MD, MPH, FAAP, is Professor and Head of the Division of Health Policy at The Johns Hopkins University School of Hygiene and Public Health, Baltimore, Maryland. Trained in Pediatrics and Epidemiology, she now devotes her energy to health services research and its translation into health policy at the local, state, and national levels. Her primary research interests are in primary care measurement, the quality of care, health status measurement (particularly for children), and child health policy. Dr. Starfield is a member of the Institute of Medicine and chairperson of the Health Services Developmental Grants Review Section of the National Center for Health Services Research, and the chairperson of the Council on Research of the American Academy of Pediatrics.

Moira Stewart, Ph.D., is Associate Professor in the Centre for Studies in Family Medicine, the Department of Family Medicine at The University of Western Ontario, London, Ontario, Canada. With a Ph.D. in Epidemiology, she has conducted research in the primary care setting for the past 15 years, addressing such topics as research methods, quality of care, doctor-patient communication in relation to outcomes, and the association of stress with health. She has published papers in *Social Science and Medicine, The Journal of the Royal College of General Practitioners, Family Practice: An International Journal,* the *Canadian Medical Association Journal,* and *Medical Care.* She recently edited a book, titled *Communicating with Medical Patients,* published by Sage Publications.

Fred Tudiver, MD, CCFP, is Assistant Professor in the Department of Family and Community Medicine, the Sunnybrook Health Science Centre and the University of Toronto, Toronto, Ontario, Canada. Born and educated in Montreal, Dr. Tudiver received his BSc at McGill University, and his MD from Memorial University in Newfoundland in 1973. He completed his family practice training at the University of Western Ontario in 1975, practiced in London until 1979, and returned to Newfoundland for a five-year stay as an assistant professor at Memorial University. He has been at Sunnybrook and the University of Toronto since 1984. His research interests include the application of self-help and mutual group support for changing lifestyles; widowerhood; and physicians' detection and management of wife assault.

DATE DUE

OC 12 '97			